What people a1

The Way of Re

Teachings of

This book is a masterpiece. Frans Stiene has brilliantly synthesized with clarity and simplicity the essence of the system of Reiki as a path of self-cultivation (shugyo) toward self-realization. The content conveys a depth of understanding of Reiki in the context of Japanese culture, arts, philosophy, and religions as a whole in a style that is engaging and illuminating. This is the kind of book one can read many times and still find deep insights into the nature of life, the universe, and being human. It is a must for Reiki teachers and practitioners as well as for those interested in exploring healing through body/mind unity, an essential concept in the Japanese arts and ways.
– **Veronique Frede**, Reiki teacher at the Japanese Culture Center in Chicago

Frans is a teacher of teachers. He provides a crystal clear bridge for Western minds to journey into the true depth of the traditional Japanese Reiki teachings. He has devoted many years to understanding Mikao Usui's perspective when he created the system of Reiki with dedication to his own practice which truly shines through his writing. Frans shows us that the true riches in the system are not in its external expression as commonly practiced, but in the internal unveiling of our True Self which naturally heals and illuminates the world around us. In my opinion, Frans is the most influential teacher living in the West and each visit to his work inspires me further. *The Way of Reiki* shines a bright light on the beautiful path to rediscover the light within each of us – it's a guide to embrace ourselves (and each other) as the vastly beautiful Universe. I'm so grateful for

his work!
– **Brighitta Moser-Clark**, author of *The Reiki Way*

I loved reading *The Way of Reiki: The Inner Teachings of Mikao Usui* by Frans Stiene! A must-read for the Global Reiki Community! Frans is living and experiencing what he is writing about and because of that his writings have a deep resonance. It is like a fresh mountain stream rippling through... bringing clarity and nourishment to everything it touches. Deeply grateful for Frans' writings and teachings; they have helped me to glimpse the deeper layers of the system of Reiki and inspire me to dig deeper into the practice. Thank you, Frans Stiene, for this incredible book. I am sure to read it again and again.
– **Maria Kammerer**, founder of Attune: The Art of Reiki and Be the Light podcast

Writing about the "why" and "how" we practice the system of Reiki seems like a simple proposition. But like the system itself, it's a deceptively simple one. It takes an immense depth of practice and understanding to explore these subjects and write such an illuminating book as *The Way of Reiki*. In short, it takes Frans Stiene, who has combined thorough research of Mikao Usui's teaching with relentless spiritual practice. Stiene is not distracted by hand-positions or technique details. Instead, he goes straight for the heart of Reiki: the state of mind in which we practice to rediscover our true self. Through every word in this book, he shines his great bright light so we can find ours.
– **Nathalie Jaspar**, author of *Reiki as a Spiritual Practice: an illustrated guide* and the *Reiki Healing Handbook*

Softening the Western veils around Reiki, this is a must-read for all practitioners of the beautiful system! Frans reveals the true nature of Reiki, which when understood and practiced diligently is much more than a hands on/off energy healing technique.

Frans simplifies the complexities of inner teachings, by first emphasizing attention given to the foundation of practice. This book is clear and systematic, encouraging readers to engage in their own direct experience, thus touching the Way of Reiki, and ultimately revealing their own true nature.

– **Yolanda Williams**, host of Reiki Radio podcast

Frans Stiene is a great teacher of the system of Reiki and a shining, fun light in the world. His new book, *The Way of Reiki*, is excellent for those who are interested in the system of Reiki and willing and wanting to explore it as part of a spiritual practice. I am grateful for Frans' teachings which always underline the interconnectedness of all things, which has brought might to my own path. I am further delighted for this new addition to the wisdom he shares so lovingly with the world, which clarifies what the world would keep hidden.

– **Kathryn Hudson**, Reiki Master Teacher, and author of *Inviting Angels into Your Life* and *Discover Your Crystal Family*

I have no doubt that Frans' new book, *The Way of Reiki*, is a true gift to the world; he is an incredible writer and wise teacher. In this book, Frans shares deep wisdom and knowledge that is easy for the reader to understand and digest. I am excited to soak up this book in its entirety and deepen my practice.

– **Jasmin Harsono**, author of *Self Reiki: Tune in to Your Life Force to Achieve Harmony and Balance*

Before I met Frans Stiene personally, we had some time of professional exchange via e-mails. Frans not only teaches Reiki and writes about it, Frans lives Reiki. The depth of his knowledge and the perseverance in his continuous practice impressed me. In my personal acquaintance I then experienced him as an extremely lively, very funny, always joking person. Quite different from what I had imagined. For me, Frans is a great example that deep spirituality and lust for life, both in distinct forms, do not have to be opposites. Spirituality does not mean a departure from the worldly or a retreat into another world. Neither does it mean that Frans' students have to evolve from intro- to extroverted people. Frans' teaching – as I got to know in his trainings and retreats, as well as in his books – runs through a common thread: it is about rediscovering one's True Self.

Every person has his personality, his aspects, which want to find expression but often cannot. They are covered with layers of experience, imprints, even programming. Thus Frans shows us what his understanding of the teachings and precepts of the Reiki founder Mikao Usui is: not only the curing of countless diseases and secret method of inviting happiness, but a guide to our True Self, which then also wants to be lived.

In this new book, *The Way of Reiki: The Inner Teachings of Mikao Usui*, Frans looks at these signposts and this path from a different viewing, from a Japanese perspective. The basics of practice are considered in the same weight as the implementation in the three Reiki levels. In my opinion, the book is not only suitable for beginners of the Reiki practice, but is also really worthwhile for long-term practitioners, as it once again stresses focus on the essentials. I wish Frans every success with his felicitous works and the book a great deal of dissemination.
– **Oliver Drewes**, author, publisher – Holistika and Reiki teacher

In his new book, *The Way of Reiki*, Frans Stiene shows us the many layers of Mikao Usui's teachings. It's written in an understandable and clear way through which he is encouraging us to Walk The Way of Reiki.
– **Helen Galpin**, co-founder of The British School of Meditation

After a journey through a jungle of doubts, fears and misunderstandings, I may realize that the impassibility exists only in my mind. But now my way has surfaced under my feet through reading *The Way of Reiki*. I finally feel in a state of deep trust and connectivity and I see myself in great shape on the way I am willing to go. Compassion is the star that is leading me. The requirement to recognize my own inner journey with and by Reiki as the foundation of a Reiki practitioner and teacher, I see confirmed in Frans' book *The Way of Reiki*. With absolute comprehensibility Frans once again illustrates in a clear manner how to discover and live our True Self, and his authenticity in "Being Reiki" manifests itself once again in this book. He empowers us, he invites us to go on the way of fully recognizing, appreciating, and respecting ourselves. We are encouraged to realize our oneness with everything, step by step, by continuous practice and to spread this realization – especially as Reiki practitioners as well as teachers. Frans' book teaches us to express the essence of "Being Reiki" in words. *The Way of Reiki* is in my eyes a wonderful must-have.

– **Claudia Kindereit**, vice-president of Reiki-Verband Germany

In his book, *The Way of Reiki*, Frans Stiene has grounded the system of Reiki solidly as a Japanese practice, art and way of life. Thoroughly researched and deeply understood, the pages of this book share gems that you can take away to support a clearer and cleaner practice.

– **Bronwen Logan (Stiene)**, coauthor of *The Reiki Sourcebook*, *Your Reiki Treatment*, and *The Japanese Art of Reiki*

I have known Frans Stiene on a professional and personal level for over fifteen years. His love for and commitment to Reiki and the System of Reiki, his diligence and commitment to research together with his willingness to share this research and knowledge is a great service to the Reiki Community. Reiki is first and foremost a Spiritual Practice and is the foundation stone that all Reiki teachings are based on. In his latest book, *The Way of Reiki: The Inner Teachings of Mikao Usui*,

Frans expands on this fact with clarity and in a way that is easy for readers to understand. He outlines how to rediscover and to be at one with our True Self, rather than living in duality and to recognise that Reiki is more than a hands on/off energy healing technique. There are so many positive passages in this book that I could write a book on how important I believe it is for all Reiki Practitioners and Teachers to read it.

– **John Coleman**, president of Australian Reiki Connection Inc., the Association of Australia Reiki Professionals

I am a Tendai monk. The founder of Tendai Sect, Denkyo Daishi Saicho, stressed Doshin – Heart for the way – as of most importance. In Denjyutsu Isshin Kaimon, Kojo (Tendai monk 779-858) quotes Saicho's famous words: "There is livelihood in Doshin, there is Doshin in livelihood." I have had the opportunity to work with Frans Stiene upon his visits to Japan, when I had the honor of guiding him through Buddhist practices. I was thoroughly impressed with Frans' Doshin and was struck with awe. In high regards to Frans Stiene's Doshin, I have presented him with the Kesa – monk's stole – which I received upon initiation to priesthood. Kesa is the soul of a priest. Having witnessed his Doshin and soul, both in person and through his books, I look forward to Frans' further endeavors. Reiki is not merely a "technique", but has a vital role in guiding one to reach "perfection as a human being". The idea contained in the precepts, "just for today, do not anger, do not worry…" also is reflected in One Day, One Life by my teacher, Sakai Yusai Dai Ajari. If you want to know whether a teacher is a true Reiki teacher or not, all you have to do is to ask him what the true self is. Without the trustworthy insight of the true self, nobody can insist he is a true disciple of Mikao Usui. His books testify that the author is one of the true Reiki teachers.

– **Takeda Hakusai Ajari**

I'm interested and impressed by Reiki and have very positive feelings about it. I think I find it almost mystical.

– **John Cleese**, comedian, author, actor, producer and screenwriter

Of Frans Stiene's many invaluable books on Reiki, The Way of Reiki is the crown jewel.

After training with Frans across thirteen Shinpiden Reiki training workshops and intensive Reiki retreats, reading the hundreds of posts about Reiki from his blog and social media channels, and discussing innumerable topics on e-mail and in-person with Frans, I have had the good fortune to get an appreciation of the depth of the system of Reiki.

Somehow Frans has done the impossible. He has packed all these teachings, great insights, and then some more into this fabulous offering, The Way of Reiki.

Establishing the non-dual essence of the teachings in the system of Reiki, Frans leads the serious practitioner into realizing that the system of Reiki has been, is, and will remain a path to Self-realization at its core.

If you are a sincere spiritual seeker, or a current Reiki practitioner or Reiki teacher, you are in for a great treat with this book. The Way of Reiki doesn't just show you clearly the non-dual essence of Reiki, it points you clearly to the Great Bright Light that is your own real nature. It is a resounding reminder that you are Reiki.

– **Sundar Kadayam**, founder of ReikiHealingNetwork.com, author of *Awaken: An Experiential Exploration of Enlightenment*

In sixteen sweet and deeply profound chapters, plus a not-to-skip Appendix, Frans Stiene holds our hands on a deep dive into the Buddhist, Taoist, and Shinto philosophical and cultural frameworks and contexts through which Mikao Usui developed the teachings and practices of Usui Reiki Ryoho. Through the chapters, Frans weaves a strand of thinking, practice, and being that grows into a beautifully textured tapestry. By the end of The Way of Reiki, this tapestry reveals the most significant warp and weft of the practice of the system of Reiki. What is revealed? That through a commitment to practicing the elements in the system of Reiki we can rest the mind in non-duality, in our innate spaciousness, and over time, experience freedom and peace. A must-read for students and practitioners of any spiritual tradition of wisdom and compassion.

– **Elise M. Brenner**, PhD, Brenner Reiki Healing, author of *Reiki: A Self-Practice To Live in Peace with Self and Others*

Frans Stiene takes us deeper into the healing Art of Usui Reiki Ryôhô, in his new book The Way of Reiki, by drawing on the teachings of Mikao Usui, traditional Japanese esoteric practices, and teachings of that time.

Combining these with his own direct experience, Frans eloquently lays bare for us the essence of the system of Reiki and our pathway to our true nature, inviting us to push the boundaries of our own practice.

An essential read for any Reiki teacher or student wishing to access the deepest-most healings of the system of Reiki, for the benefit of humanity and our planet.

– **Mary Hambly**, editor of The Reiki News, New Zealand

The Way of Reiki -
The Inner Teachings
of Mikao Usui

The Way of Reiki - The Inner Teachings of Mikao Usui

Frans Stiene

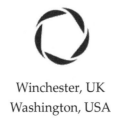

Winchester, UK
Washington, USA

JOHN HUNT PUBLISHING

First published by O-Books, 2022
O-Books is an imprint of John Hunt Publishing Ltd., 3 East St., Alresford,
Hampshire SO24 9EE, UK
office@jhpbooks.com
www.johnhuntpublishing.com
www.o-books.com

For distributor details and how to order please visit the 'Ordering' section on our website.

Design: Matthew Greenfield

UK: Printed and bound by CPI Group (UK) Ltd, Croydon, CR0 4YY
Printed in North America by CPI GPS partners

We operate a distinctive and ethical publishing philosophy in
all areas of our business, from our global network of authors to
production and worldwide distribution.

Contents

Other titles by this author

The Inner Heart of Reiki: Rediscovering Your True Self
ISBN: 978 1 78535 055 9

Reiki Insights
ISBN: 978 1 78535 735 0

With Bronwen Stiene

A–Z of Reiki Pocketbook: Everything About Reiki
ISBN: 978 1 90504 789 5

The Japanese Art of Reiki
ISBN: 978 1 90504 702 9

The Reiki Sourcebook
ISBN: 978 1 84694 181 8

Your Reiki Treatment
ISBN: 978 1 84694 013 2

Thank you, Eukie, my mum, and thank you, Oliver Stiene, for being great teachers in my life.

In our lifetime we must grab hold of the True Self. We have to discover our true purpose. Arriving at this True Self is what we call enlightenment. Truly seeing ourselves, keeping our feet firmly planted on the ground, we walk this way without losing sight of who we are. That is attaining the Way.

– Discovering the True Self by Kōdō Sawaki

Foreword

In Japanese, "way" or *Dō* has connotations of philosophy and doctrine. It also intrinsically implies the concept of discipline. Through repeated practice, we gain a deep understanding and mastery of a subject, of our mind, and the mysteries of life.

When I first learned the system of Reiki, I was not taught a "way". I was taught a bunch of definitions, tools, and techniques with very little explanation. I was told where to place my hands and how long, but never why or in what state of mind. When I finished my Reiki 2 training, I performed Reiki sessions – performed being the key word. There was no depth, just lots of guesswork and fear, "Am I doing this right? Is this doing anything?"

It wasn't until I came across a book written by Frans Stiene that it dawned on me that there was a lot more depth to the Reiki system than I credited it. So, when I trained with him for the first time, I got the most valuable teaching in my practice: the Reiki system is not something to be performed but to be explored.

Frans didn't teach me more tools or techniques. Instead, he taught me why we practice and from what state of mind we practice. He taught me that understanding trumps techniques, even if this understanding is often born out of repeating a technique with discipline.

The Way of Reiki now brings this gift to every Reiki practitioner. In this jewel of a book, Frans conveys the wisdom acquired during years of serious practice and learning in an accessible way for each level of Reiki practice.

Frans brings to life the Reiki precepts both as the core of the system and its ultimate goal: to embody them. He unlocks the hidden meanings of the Reiki kanji and symbols, so they become more than tools. He shifts the way we think about attunements and hands-on healing by giving us the historical and spiritual context from which they were born.

In short, he gives us the ultimate roadmap to understanding the teachings of Mikao Usui and points us towards rediscovering our True Self.

– Nathalie Jaspar, author of *Reiki as a Spiritual Practice: an illustrated guide* and the *Reiki Healing Handbook*

New York, May 12, 2021

Preface

Out of the well of my practice this book emerged. It came up like a flash of lightning and also was suddenly written like a lightning flash, illuminating my own personal practice. Therefore, writing this book has deepened my own understanding of the system of Reiki as a whole. While the system of Reiki is beautiful in its simplicity, the inner teachings of Mikao Usui are not easy to understand. Yet Mikao Usui made it easy for us and for that I am grateful. I would not be able to write this book without the profound teachings of Mikao Usui.

And neither would I have been able to write this book without the profound teachings of many other masters. Yes, I write the word masters here, because I believe these are real masters. The first I would like to thank is my teacher Takeda Hakusai Ajari, whose own direct experience is steeped in dedicated practices. He is a wonderful teacher and a great example for me to sit on my butt and do the practices so that I can have a direct experience not just once, but hopefully many times. The diligent practice that he inspires flows into a continuous experience in all I do.

There are many other teachers who have helped me with this book. To honor them I have peppered the book with quotes from those who have taught me. Not all in person – some through their writings and teachings which, after having read their books, left me with a deeper understanding and insight. I am forever grateful for these kinds of teachers to have appeared on my path.

My mum Eukie and Oliver Stiene are also among those wonderful teachers who have shown me that we have to be more open-minded and natural in all we do. I thank you both from the bottom of my essence for being in my life and sharing this journey with me. I want to thank my editor Carol Ryan who really understands what I am trying to say even if my writing is all over the place. And of course the publishing team has my gratitude for being so wonderful and accommodating.

There are many more, people I meet randomly on the street who offer a small sentence here and there which triggers an insight, and of course all the people who come and join me for courses. I don't really see them as students, rather I see them as friends. We are all friends holding each other's hands, together walking the way home to our True Self.

Your real self is a kind of energy. It is the original energy, which is constantly arising at the very incipient moment. At the very incipient moment, there is no "I." There is nothing to call "I" because there is no perception of "I." There is no "who." There is nothing to call "who" because you realize there is no existence to attach to as your own. At that time you are simultaneously this very moment itself, extending into every inch of the universe.
– The Light That Shines Through Infinity by Dainin Katagiri

Usui Reiki Ryôhô as Taught by The International House of Reiki

Nowadays there are many people teaching Usui Reiki Ryôhô. But what is the difference among these, and what does the International House of Reiki teach?

I first learned the system of Reiki in 1999; the way I was taught was a very modern way. I longed for more and believed that there were elements missing in what I was taught. So after some exploration I took a Shinpiden Reiki III course with a teacher in Japan in 2001. Those teachings did not satisfy my thirst for a deeper understanding of Mikao Usui's teachings so I kept exploring. In 2003 I took another Shinpiden Reiki III course in Japan. But again my thirst for a deeper understanding of Mikao Usui's teachings was not quenched. While I got something from each learning experience, I still felt something was missing.

Each time I felt there were things missing: practices, teachings, experiences not internalized. Yes, they talked about it, but the real deeper practices were not really emphasized or taught.

So I kept exploring and practicing myself.

I wanted to learn what Mikao Usui was practicing himself. What was his background, and where did the tools come from that he taught in the system of Reiki? I wanted to go to the source so to speak and not get sidetracked with other teachings that came from Chūjirō Hayashi who, as Hiroshi Doi and Hyakuten Inamoto had already pointed out through their research, had changed Mikao Usui's teachings in some ways.

Mikao Usui sat on Mount Kurama for 21 days – not a simple task, and he was not camping either. He was practicing specific meditations to let his ego die, so to speak.

Through more and more research I discovered that Mikao Usui had taken some of his teachings from the esoteric Japanese

Buddhist tradition. So I started to explore these.

In 2012 I was lucky enough to be invited by an Ajari in Japan. An Ajari is a priest who can train other priests. The first time I went to train with Takeda Hakusai, I stayed at his temple for a week for one-on-one training; this training was challenging, from 4am in the morning till about 11pm at night. He pushed me, challenged me, taught me, and finally I found what I was looking for. A deeper understanding of Mikao Usui's teachings, I was home. Since then I have worked with Takeda Ajari to explore myself and the deeper elements of the system of Reiki. In 2019 some of the International House of Reiki students were able to meet with Takeda Ajari in Japan and received teachings and blessings from him. Over the next few years, Takeda Ajari and I hope to slowly help people to explore more about their own True Self and the esoteric elements of the system of Reiki.

So what we teach at the International House of Reiki is unique, as we focus on the esoteric elements of the system of Reiki to help you gain a deeper understanding of your True Self. In this book, I aim to introduce you to some of these teachings. It is not a replacement for a class, but I hope it will add to your knowledge and open some doors in your mind and to your True Self. Our learning and exploration never stops, and so we walk with each other hand in hand the road to self-empowerment.

Every day, all you have to do is stand up in emptiness, open your heart, and accept the lively energy of your life. Then you are ready to act based on wisdom.
– The Light That Shines Through Infinity by Dainin Katagiri

Introduction

I start with the quote below to indicate that there is so much more to the system of Reiki than the standard teachings taught and practiced these days.

When John studied with Takata, he made over 20 audio tapes of her lectures and classes. On one of the tapes she discusses travelling to Japan in order to teach her approach to Reiki. While there, she met some Japanese citizens who were actively practicing and preserving Reiki as they understood in Japan. Takata regarded their approach as entirely valid, but inappropriate for the West. It was highly complex, required years of training and was closely intertwined with religious practices. She felt these factors would deter students in the West and hobble the spread of Reiki through the world at a time when, in her view, it was urgently needed.
– Hand to Hand by John Harvey Gray

Mrs. Takata was influential in bringing the system of Reiki to the West after she had trained in Japan. However, as we can see from the above statement, Mrs. Takata discovered when she went back to Japan that the system of Reiki as practiced there was very different than what she had learned from Chūjirō Hayashi. And as most of the teachings from Japan come through Chūjirō Hayashi, we have a very different understanding of what Mikao Usui really intended to practice and teach. In a way this is not bad at all; we have to start somewhere. But to really gain a deep understanding of Mikao Usui's teachings, we have to investigate what he was really pointing out. The statement above notes that the Japanese application of Mikao Usui's teachings was highly complex, required years of training and was closely intertwined with religious practices. These religious practices are esoteric Japanese Buddhism, Zen, Shugendo, and

Shinto. But that doesn't mean we have to become a Buddhist, or abandon our own faith traditions, in order to embrace the way of Reiki as originally intended.

It only means that Mikao Usui had rediscovered our buddha nature as the main focus point of his practice. This is also why he himself went to Mount Kurama to practice a specific 21 day meditation practice. These practices are still being done within Japanese esoteric traditions and are not easy. They are not done to rediscover hands on/off healing; they are done to lay bare our True Self and this is what Mikao Usui based his teachings on. Thus we go back to the roots of his instructions and practices. There's no need to invent something new; his teachings are perfect the way they are.

This is also why in 2012, I started to train with Japanese priest Takeda Hakusai Ajari. I wanted to see what Mrs. Takata saw when she went back to Japan and rediscovered how the system of Reiki was practiced traditionally in Japan. *The Way of Reiki* is about this journey, which in fact started much earlier than 2012. To be precise, in 1999 I first stepped on the path of spiritual awakening. So far this has been a wonderful journey full of ups and downs, and so rewarding.

The book begins with how to prepare ourselves to be able to practice well. These are important instructions and often not taught within the wider Reiki community. But as we will discover, if we want our practice to bear fruit, to reveal what Mikao Usui indicated in his teachings, Satori – spiritual awakening, or in Japan sometimes called anshin ritsumei – peaceful mind, we need to have fertile ground. That means we have to prepare the ground, the foundation.

Satori isn't arriving at a special place that is difficult to reach; it is simply being natural.
– Discovering the True Self by Kōdō Sawaki

After we have prepared the ground and laid a solid foundation, we can start to do the meditation practices as taught within the traditional system of Reiki. To get the most out of our practice, we cannot only learn from a book, but also will want to find a qualified teacher who can help us to prepare the foundation and teach the practices according to their own direct experience. A teacher of most benefit will be one who points us not to duality but to our True Self, our non-dual nature. Why non-duality? Because non-duality is what Mikao Usui pointed out and it is only through the direct experience of this in our own mind and body that we create a peaceful environment for ourselves and others. And this is so needed in our modern world today.

Dualism has to be thrown away as well, or society cannot be truly liberated.
– Ten Ox Herding Pictures by Zen Master Shodo Harada

Part I:
Preparation

Before we practice, we have to prepare. Just like when we start to grow a tomato plant, first we have to prepare the soil, pick the right spot, and create the right environment for the plant to grow and thrive. Without the right environment the plant will not bear any fruit. Or it may bear fruit that is not too healthy or is not the size, shape or taste that we were aiming for. This is why within this book we start with exploring the preparation practices, so that we create the right environment. This in turn will give us the right fruit of our practice.

Chapter 1:

Reiki

When we put a name on that energy, it is called Buddha, buddha-nature, or real self. We use different terms, but each one means the same original energy of the whole world, the boundless and compassionate energy of being, which is constantly coming up from deep on the ground like spring water.
– The Light That Shines Through Infinity by Dainin Katagiri

So what is Reiki? Literally the word Reiki translates as spiritual energy. This is not some kind of specific vibration which hangs somewhere in the sky and needs to be pulled into our body to channel it. This spiritual energy is our essence, our True Self, or as my teacher Takeda Ajari says, Reiki is Kami and Buddha. Kami in Japan stands for our own inner divine being and Buddha is our buddha nature. But these are just names. In essence, how can you point out your True Self which is so vast and so open, which has no beginning and end? Impossible.

Thus we have to say something so that we make it workable. Mikao Usui, the founder of the system of Reiki, called this spiritual energy not only Reiki but also Great Bright Light 大光明 dai kômyô. Why, because our True Self is luminous and shines out through the whole universe; in fact it is the universe. Or as the ancient teachers used to say, we are the universe and the universe is us. It is our non-dual nature, or as they point out in the Japanese teachings, dai kômyô is emptiness.

What we call the source of human personality – the True Self – is said to be this kind of eternal existence, yet it does not exist outside the living body.
– Introduction to Zen Training: A Physical Approach to Meditation

and Mind-Body Training by Omori Sogen

Often we get confused by these names if we do not have the right understanding. For example, when we talk about emptiness we might think this means that we are empty like zombies, that our lives will become boring because we are empty. But this is of course a big misunderstanding; emptiness is like light, luminous, which means we see everything clearly. We can see, for example, why and when we get angry which in turn gives us the possibility to let the anger just melt away. And through this clarity we also see how we can help others, how we can be compassionate to others and to ourselves. Because the essence of emptiness is compassion and wisdom – clarity. But not only that – it is pure energy, unpolluted by our confused and mistaken views.

In other words, we can say that emptiness – Reiki – is a state of mind in which we have not put extra ideas in our mind, ideas that may come from experiences or judgements rather than from our True Self, our buddha nature. Emptiness is a state of no borders – no expectations, no labels, no preconceived ideas, no mistaken beliefs, unfabricated, of just pure freedom, which is wide open, and free from dual fixation. And with this emptiness, pure energy flows through our whole being, within and out like a great bright light emanating its radiance in all directions. This pure energy is our driving force for compassion and kindness, our motivation to help others, and help others to rediscover their own great bright light. This is Reiki.

Originally we are completely vastness. In the vastness of the universe, there is no dichotomy, no discrimination; there is perfect peace and harmony. Philosophically speaking, this is called emptiness. Sometimes vastness is personalized, and it's called Buddha. If you experience that emptiness, it is called buddha-

nature. Plainly speaking, it is universal consciousness.
– The Light That Shines Through Infinity by Dainin Katagiri

This emptiness – non-duality – is our birthright, this is our humanness. Often we get confused and think that being human must mean being angry and worried, at least some if not all of the time. But according to the Online Etymology Dictionary (www.etymonline.com), the word "human" came from old French (humain) and Latin (humanus) meaning "of man", but also meaning "humane, philanthropic, kind, gentle, polite; learned, refined, civilized". As we can see from this perspective, being human means being kind, gentle, and polite. Thus if we are angry, worried, and fearful we lose this kindness, gentleness, and politeness and in fact we are the opposite of being human! Hence the system of Reiki helps us to become a true human being again, full of love and compassion.

Usui Sensei taught that practices which are based on the correct understanding of nature and the universe help develop the self. When Reiki practitioners come to a full understanding of such practices and are able to discipline themselves, their speech and conduct fall into alignment with the universe and they attain infinitive power. This is what it means to be a true human being.
– from 会員のみに配布する霊気療法のしおり Leaflet of Reiki Ryôhô – Members Only, translation found in Hiroshi Doi's manual

Thus to be able to realize that we are Reiki, that we are non-duality, emptiness, a great bright light, buddha, kami, the universe, or whatever word you want to use, we need to have a system in place to help us remember this. Because remembering this as we live in modern society is not so easy. This is why Mikao Usui placed very specific practices within his system. However, we need to practice them in the correct way, just like making a cake. For example, if we bake a cake and we put the ingredients together in the wrong way or we do not read the instructions correctly or do not use the correct time and temperature, we get a cake which might not even be edible.

Therefore we need a qualified teacher who has walked the path themselves so that they can guide the student the right way to practice the system of Reiki, so that the student can have a direct experience of their True Self, of their non-dual nature. Because it is only through this direct experience that we are really creating a difference in the world, creating it in ourselves. And that is what the system of Reiki is all about. We will start to get a much clearer perception of this as we explore in this book all the different teachings Mikao Usui placed within his system. We also will start to discover that the system of Reiki is so much more than the commonly promoted component of hands on/off healing. That is one component of it yes, but there is so much more to discover.

To know our True Self is the basis of our own being. If we realize this fact, we cannot afford to do anything before we solve this problem of knowing our True Selves.
– Introduction to Zen Training: A Physical Approach to Meditation and Mind-Body Training by Omori Sogen

Chapter 2:

The System of Reiki

To lay bare our non-dual nature – Reiki – we need to practice the system of Reiki; hence we have Reiki and the System of Reiki. To do this we have to go within, within our own mind, body, and energy, pointing inwards as all the teachers of old did. But in modern days we have started to look more and more outside of ourselves, therefore stepping away from truly rediscovering our True Self. Our True Self can only be truly rediscovered when we stop looking outside of ourselves and bring all the practices within. Mikao Usui pointed this out again and again in his own teachings as we will see in our exploration of the different practices and pointers within the system of Reiki.

There is no difference in the ways of the ancients and the ways of today.
– Discovering the True Self by Kōdō Sawaki

The system of Reiki consists of 5 elements; we will explore these to their fullest so that we can get a very clear idea what Mikao Usui's teachings are all about. We also will examine how to practice so that we can lay bare our innate compassion and wisdom.

Something that works is using energy. From ancient times, people in the East have developed spiritual, medical, and martial art traditions based on the flow of universal energy as the life force called chi, qi, or ki.
– The Light That Shines Through Infinity by Dainin Katagiri

The first element is the precepts: they are the base of the whole system. If we want to build a house, we start with the foundation. This needs to be strong and solid, else the whole house will collapse. Although they are the foundation of the system, in many modern Reiki teachings the precepts are only touched upon briefly, which creates an unstable foundation. When we come to the deeper practices, we might not be able to progress because our base is not solid enough. Therefore it is best to take your time with understanding each element. What does taking the time mean? It means practicing and contemplating the practices and teachings again and again and again, over and over.

Traditionally your teacher would guide you in this and only let you take the next step when they thought you were ready, that your foundation was strong enough. But these days we want to rush through these teachings, tick a box and quickly become a teacher. By doing that we miss the juicy parts of the teachings and of course we also will miss the direct experience of our True Self. It will become impossible to lay bare our essential nature, emptiness. Emptiness is like a mirror. A mirror reflects everything but the mirror never clings, labels, wants, or judges; it is free. And our human journey on this planet is to truly embrace this freedom. Therefore, take your time with each of these elements because it is only through having the direct experience again and again that we can bring it into our daily life, in all we do. This is compassion to yourself.

The second element is a set of very specific meditation practices which work with breath, our energy, and the art of gaining control over our monkey mind. These practices are about gaining focus so that we do not get distracted by all our senses, by what we see, hear, feel, taste and smell. It is through this non-distraction that we can lay bare our non-dual nature, our essence. Again this is going inwards, in our own body, because the body is the house of the mind and of the energy and it is within the body that our traumas are stored. This can stop the flow of our energy, which in turn can create illnesses and confusion. But these meditation practices also need to be practiced again and again, preferably on a daily basis, not just once, or twice, but maybe for years and years. Since our "goal" so to speak is to lay bare our True Self, why stop halfway? Keep practicing until you lay bare your True Self to its fullest, its complete awakening, its complete self-illumination.

The third element is hands on/off healing: first on ourselves. And only when we have gained a deep understanding, a solid foundation, can we start to practice this aspect of the teachings on others. Often we want to jump straight into helping others, but if our minds are still confused how can we truly help others? Therefore it is better to first gain a good understanding, intellectually, about the teachings and have the direct experience of what it means to have a good foundation before we venture into helping others. Else it will be like the blind leading the blind.

The fourth element is symbols and mantras, which start to be taught within Okuden Reiki II and Shinpiden Reiki III. These symbols and mantras also have to be internalized; they are like keys to unlock what is hidden inside of us, our great bright light, our True Self. This is why Mikao Usui called the second level of his teachings Okuden, which means hidden or inner teachings. It points directly to where we have to focus: not outside but inside our own mind, body, and energy. And through focusing inside we start to find out what is hidden within, waiting to be uncovered. If we use the symbols and mantras externally, it will be hard to lay bare our inner hidden qualities of compassion and wisdom. This is also why Mikao Usui called his third level Shinpiden. Shinpiden means mystery teachings; at this level we begin to lay bare the mystery of who we truly are, of what we all have been looking for in our life. Although often promoted as such, this level is not about teaching at all. Teaching comes from laying bare what we truly are: a great bright light, luminosity.

The fifth element is the reiju, often called initiation or attunement. But in Japan there is just one word for this ritual:

reiju, which translates as spiritual blessing or offering. In a way we also can call this fifth element the first element, but we will come back to that later. These elements are all interlinked with each other and not separate entities. All need to be practiced for us to gain a proper understanding about the system of Reiki and to have a direct experience, again and again, of our True Self. Or in other words, all five elements create a house; if one is missing or misunderstood the house might not have a roof or a back wall, for example. Hence these elements are building blocks which need to be used in the proper way and in the proper manner.

Dhammapada says,
By oneself evil is done;
By oneself one suffers.
By oneself evil is undone,
No one can purify another.
– Hakuin on Kensho by Albert Low

Chapter 3:

The Inner Meaning of Reiki

We have looked at Reiki and the system of Reiki. So now let's look a little deeper into the essence of the kanji of Reiki and what Mikao Usui was pointing out to us in it. Through looking at what Reiki is, what the system of Reiki stands for and the deeper element of the kanji of Reiki, we gain a much better understanding of what our practice is about and also how to practice.

Let's first look at the surface meaning of each kanji:

Some translations of the word Rei: 靈

* Spirit
* Life
* Soul
* Inconceivable spiritual ability
* Bright
* Unpolluted
* Pure
* Divine
* Mysterious
* Spirit; the spiritual aspect of the human being

Some translations of the word Ki: 気

* Mind
* Spirit
* Breath
* Energy
* Air
* Invisible life-force

* Vital energy connected to the breath
* Steam

So when we look at these two together we can come up with many different translations. I personally like this one: inconceivable spiritual ability of the mind. What is this inconceivable spiritual ability of the mind? It is our buddha nature, non-duality, emptiness, Kami, the great bright light, our True Self: all different words for one and the same thing. And it also points to the mind as it is the mind which experiences anshin ritsumei, peace of mind.

Now let's look at the inner meaning of the kanji of Reiki. Each kanji is made up of different elements.

Rei 靈 is made up out of
雨 and 口 and
巫雨 rain
口 mouth 巫 shaman

So the kanji of Rei 靈 tells us that a shaman is performing a ritual to let it rain, and this rain falls in three mouths. These three mouths stand for sanmitsu – the 3 mysteries of mind-body-energy. But this rain is not the typical rain we would think of. This is the spiritual rain which always falls down; it is universal rain! And the essence of the spiritual rain is emptiness – non-duality.

Ask yourself, how do you touch the universe? To touch the universe you do not have to do anything as we are so intertwined with it, it is touching us inside, outside and in between. Hence this means that it is always raining spiritual energy, which in turn means that there is no on and off for healing to take place. However, we often carry the umbrella of fear, anger, worry, attachments, and all sorts of other emotions and conditions. Often we are so busy carrying this umbrella we do not realize that the potential for healing is always there. Thus the shaman/ practitioner practices a ritual so that they can realize that it is always raining universal rain, and this rain nurtures the mind, body, energy of the practitioner. The ritual helps the shaman/ practitioner to let go of the umbrella and step out into the light and realize that they are soaked in emptiness, in Reiki. When we are soaked it means that no element of our mind, body, and energy is left untouched by this emptiness, we are it, it is our essence, our True Self.

Ki 氣 is made up out of 气 and 米
气 steam or spirit 米 rice

So in the kanji of Ki 氣 we can see rice and steam. Rice is nutrition; it nourishes and nurtures us. One of my teachers once said that now it is white rice but in the past it was brown rice. What he means is that the past teachings were more nutritious, not diluted as many of them have become over time.

But we can also see steam. So now we have to ask ourselves: how do we get steam from rice? We have to cook the rice because raw rice is not so nutritious and of course it is difficult to digest. How do we cook it? We need to boil it, and so we need fire. Thus, in a hidden inner way, we can see also fire within the kanji of Ki. But where do we put the fire? Above the pot of rice or underneath it? Underneath right? Where is our own inner fire most of the time? It is in the top part of our body; check for yourself. What happens when you get angry or worried? Your face becomes red, because your fire is in the upper part of your body. Hence the kanji of Ki tells us to make sure we keep the fire in our hara, our center, just below our navel. The more we stimulate the fire in our hara, the less angry and worried we will be. So in a way the kanji of Ki shows us the right method to embody the precepts and how not to get angry and worried.

This is one of the reasons we do the deep breathing meditation practices like jōshin kokyū hō and chanting the mantras within the system of Reiki. What stimulates fire? Air. So the deep breathing stimulates our inner fire so that it can melt all our anger, fear and worry.

We are made up of about 60% water, but most of the time our water is so stuck, frozen with anger, worry and fear. The inner fire helps us to transform our frozen water into steam again so that it can flow more easily through our body. Remember steam can penetrate every single cell of your body.

... be able to melt into any situation you might enter – to be like water, which fills any container, no matter what shape the container is, rather than like ice, which can only enter a container of its own shape and otherwise is cumbersome. When we let go of our hard edges and the things we are stuck on, we become like water, able to enter anywhere, and this brings us joy when other people's joy is present. From morning until night we think only of others, of how we can help, how we can bring joy to them, without thinking of ourselves or putting ourselves first. Like a fool, we only smile and bring warmth and joy and comfort to everyone we meet; not offering difficult explanations, we simply meet everyone with this warmth.

– Ten Ox Herding Pictures by Zen Master Shodo Harada

This frozen water represents our traumas; thus to heal our traumas and to let go of them we need to go inward, in our body, as this is where the transformation takes place and where our traumas are stored. The steam becomes rain again and so the energy starts to flow more freely through our mind – body – energy. But what does this process look like: rain, steam (mist), heat...? It is nature! Look around outside. In nature we see the rain fall down, the sun heats the earth, the mist rises and it becomes rain again. An up and down movement of natural elements and energy. Our mind-body-energy is a microcosm within the macrocosm, we are the universe and the universe is us; we are nature.

This is why people like Mikao Usui went into the mountains to realize that they are nature and that this external natural process of rain, heat, steam is also an internal process. This internal process is a very important element within Mikao Usui's system. In fact we can see this internal process of rain, heat, and mist pointed out in many ancient spiritual teachings, often called inner bliss, inner joy or blazing and dripping. A good teacher can guide you through this natural process inside your body-mind-energy through teaching you the right practice at the right time. But as it is made of mist we also realize that we cannot grasp mist; we cannot hold onto it. This in itself is yet another teaching, it points to non-attachment, not holding onto the experiences. It points to the concept that these experiences are also empty in nature. Therefore just practice the right practices at the right time with the right motivation and right aim.

So if you see something wonderful don't get stuck! Accept it, experience it, and then keep your mouth shut. Your experience will never disappear. It stays with your life and penetrates your life. It's not necessary to attach to it. Let it go!
– The Light That Shines Through Infinity by Dainin Katagiri

Here is another hidden inner meaning of the kanji of Reiki. When the rain falls it doesn't judge, label, or distinguish; it is just falling, but the trees, shrubs, flowers take from it whatever they need. The mist and the sun do the same; they do not judge, label or distinguish. This is also why Mikao Usui used the kanji of Reiki to teach his students not to label, judge and distinguish when they meditate, perform a hands on healing on themselves or others, and perform a reiju.

But it is all good and well to intellectually know this; the next step is to actually create the right inner atmosphere to have a direct experience of the inner meaning of the kanji of Reiki. Through having this direct inner experience again and again we become a wonderful vehicle for these natural elements to manifest within us, which in turn creates the perfect setting for helping others, for showing compassion to ourselves and others. We also can see this pointed out within the precepts, which we will discuss in the next chapter.

Ki can be thought of as an energy that flows through the body (and through the entire universe), and it is referred to as "mind" and is centered specifically in the lower abdomen.
– The Japanese Arts and Self-Cultivation by Robert E. Carter

Chapter 4:

The Precepts

In the big scale of life, precept is the activity of the whole universe, which naturally ripens a tree's life, a person's life, and the life of all sentient beings. This is the most important meaning of precepts.
– The Light That Shines Through Infinity by Dainin Katagiri

Let's start at the beginning of all the practices... the precepts. They not only are the foundation of the system of Reiki, but they also are the outcome.

招	福	の	祕	法
shou	fuku	no	hi	hou
invite	blessings	of	secret	method

萬	病	の	靈	藥
man	byoo	no	rei	yaku
10.000	illnesses	of	spiritual	medicine

今日	丈けは	怒る な
kyo	dakewa	ikaru na
Today	only	anger not

心配 すな	感謝 して
Shinpai suna	kansha shite
Worry not	gratitude do

業 をはけめ	人 に	親切	に
gyo o hageme	hito ni	shinsetsu	ni
practice diligently	people to	kindness	be

朝夕
asayuu
morning and evening

合掌　して
gassho shite
gassho perform

心　に
kokoro ni
Mind to
(Keep in your mind)

念じ
nenji
pray silently

口　に
kuchi ni
mouth at

唱へ　よ
tonae yo
chant do

心身
Shinshin
Mind and body

改善
kaizen
improve

臼井靈氣療法
Usui Reiki Ryôhô

肇祖
Choso
Founder

臼井甕男
Usui Mikao
Usui Mikao

The secret method of inviting blessings
The spiritual medicine of 10.000 illnesses

Today only
Do not anger
Do not worry
Be grateful
Practice diligently – be true to your way and your being
Be kind to yourself and others – show compassion to yourself

and others

Morning and evening perform gassho
Keep in your mind
Chant with your mouth

Improve your mind-body

Usui Reiki Ryôhô
Founder
Mikao Usui

There are many different ways to translate the precepts due to kanji having different meanings. So it all depends on what kind of meaning we use during the translation and also on the translator's own spiritual insights. To give a quick example: gyo can mean work, practice, pure experience and also karma. Thus gyo o hagame can also be translated as *be true to your pure experience*, which in turn also has different layers. And therefore it often has been translated as *be true to your way and your being*. (We will explore this later.) True kindness in the case of Mikao Usui is really compassion, hence the translation of *show compassion to yourself and others*.

> *If I say, "Just be kind to others without expecting anything," and you do it, but while you are doing it, you are constantly thinking, "I must just be kind without expecting anything," then a thought is still coming up. The real meaning of "just be kind" is that finally even this thought doesn't appear. That is no-thought, we say.*
> *— The Light That Shines Through Infinity by Dainin Katagiri*

When we look at the precepts we see that there are many layers to them. We also see that they are full of teachings on how to practice the system of Reiki and what to expect on our journey.

Let us explore the precepts so that we can benefit from their teachings and instructions.

The secret method of inviting blessings is pointing to the embodiment of the precepts. Many people mistakenly believe that the blessings point towards the reiju, but this is not the case at all. The blessings mentioned in the precepts are all about the supreme embodiment of the precepts in our daily life, in all we do. Think about it: what would the most profound blessing be? A life without anger and worry in which we can be grateful, true to our way and our being and in which we have compassion to ourselves and others – or a blessing of reiju?

The spiritual medicine of 10.000 illnesses: Within Taoism and Buddhism we often see the phrase of 10.000 things, which in reality means an infinite number. Thus through the embodiment of the precepts we lay bare the spiritual medicine of infinite illnesses. We often just see the surface meaning of this, but the inner meaning is that the precepts cut through the root of all our illnesses. If we look deeply enough we can see that the precepts are a description of our True Self, which Mikao Usui pointed out within Shinpiden Reiki III as dai kômyô 大光明 the Great Bright Light. When we lay bare our True Self – emptiness – non-duality, which is the spiritual medicine, and as soon as we have laid bare the fullness of our True Self, we have cut the root of all our illnesses, of the 10.000 illnesses. And at that stage we will be free. Think about it: in that state of Great Bright Light, True Self, there is no anger, there is no worry. There is just gratefulness and being true to our way and our being, and above all there is compassion.

Compassion naturally occurs in the state of selflessness.
– Kaji: Empowerment and Healing in Esoteric Buddhism by Ryuko Oda

Thus by providing us with the precepts, Mikao Usui showed us the way towards emptiness – non-duality. And he showed us in the precepts that by laying bare this emptiness to its fullest, we will have cut the roots of all our illnesses. This in turn is the secret method of inviting blessings. Why secret? It's not secret in the sense of – shhh! – mustn't tell anyone! In fact, showing others how to lay bare their emptiness is the most compassionate thing we can do. The precepts call this method secret because our True Self is so close that often we do not see it, as instead we are busy looking outside of ourselves. But when we turn our gaze inwards, we start to discover this inner secret, the essence of our True Self. This inner secret, essence, True Self is emptiness and non-duality, which in reality cannot be divided.

Today only is used a lot within Japanese Buddhism. This phrase points towards every action we are performing today: sleeping, standing, eating, walking, working, you name it. Whatever it is, we have to infuse it with the precepts. As we have seen, the precepts are an expression of emptiness and non-duality, which means we have to infuse every action we are doing with emptiness and non-duality. But this is easier said than done. Therefore Mikao Usui also placed specific practices within his teachings to help us to have that direct experience and maintain it through every thing we do, every action we take. What are these practices? They are hands on/off healing on ourselves as an act of meditation practice, meditation practices such as jōshin kokyū hō and seishin toitsu, meditating on the symbols and mantras and the reiju, and of course the precepts themselves.

We should be able to say "every day is a good day" not only in easy or comfortable times but even in the most difficult and challenging times. When we know, no matter what comes along, that every day is a good day, that essence will extend throughout the heavens and the earth.

– Ten Ox Herding Pictures by Zen Master Shodo Harada

"Only" also stands for the transcending of time, of past, present and future within Japanese spiritual teachings.

In the same way, there is no idea of time in the world of "only."
The state of "only" transcends time.
— Introduction to Zen Training: A Physical Approach to Meditation and Mind-Body Training by Omori Sogen

Thus the more we look at the system of Reiki from a traditional Japanese perspective, we can see what Mikao Usui used as the roots for his teachings: Zen, Tendai Buddhism, Shugendo, and Shinto.

Not is an interesting element within the precepts and again the root is Japanese Buddhism.

In Buddhism we use the words no or not to show that nothing has its own separate existence, everything is interconnected and produced by interdependent co-origination.
— Each Moment is theUniverse by Dainin Katagiri

Here we can see that the word "no" or "not" points to interconnectedness. It is through interconnectedness that we get angry and worried in the first place! Anger and worry don't exist in a vacuum and don't suddenly just appear; they appear due to other interconnected elements, and if we can see this deeply, we can realize the empty nature of it. This is what "no" or "not" points out.

The negative term "no" or "not" implies transcendence of conceptual thinking coming from your human mind.
— The Light That Shines Through Infinity by Dainin Katagiri

Again Dainin Katagiri points out that we have to transcend our conceptual thinking, our confused mind to really understand why there is "no" or "not". Why? Because it points to emptiness.

Do not anger. We can write a whole book about how to deal with anger. But for now I want to go to the essence of this precept. We have to ask ourselves, who gets angry? I get angry. Then where is this I? Can we find it? Does it have a shape or color? Is this I residing in my heart or in my brain? Again and again we have to investigate the I who gets angry and the I who holds onto that anger. The more we do this, the deeper we go. And then, when we realize that the I cannot be found, we can have the direct experience of emptiness. The I is empty. This does not mean that we are zombies; this empty quality is full of compassion, wisdom, and energy. When we have that direct experience of no I, then who is there to get angry?

Normally, the way we get angry is that first a thought arises and then we cling to this thought. We label the thought and the feeling that arises in us, and we get angry. But when we are in the state of emptiness, a thought will arise but the clinging has ceased. And therefore the thought will dissipate all by itself, with no label and no judgement. Thus no anger. There are many methods we can use to stop our anger: we can focus on our breathing when we feel the thought of anger arising. But if our angry thought is too strong, just focusing on our breathing will not give the desired result, because the breath is too subtle. Hence we need to cut anger by the root, and again, what is the root? The root is the direct experience of emptiness. Then no matter what angry thought arises it will have no base to stand on because we will not cling to the thought. And hence anger will dissipate all by itself. Without this direct experience of emptiness we will never be able to dissolve our anger completely; therefore Mikao Usui pointed out again and again this necessity of the direct experience of emptiness – non-duality.

However, if, in our quiet self-reflection, we turn our mind's eye
from the external world to the internal life to realize our true self-

nature we will clearly understand that the true nature of our Self, which we thought up until now had a fixed, real existence, is in fact no self-nature. Because we have no self-nature, there is neither self nor other. In the absence of self and other, there cannot be such passions as joy, anger, sorrow, and pleasure, all of which arise from the dualities of self and other. All things, just as they are in their very essence of no self-nature, function without any hindrance in freely flowing transformation.
– Introduction to Zen Training: A Physical Approach to Meditation and Mind-Body Training by Omori Sogen

Do not worry follows the same teaching as do not anger. We have to cut worry and fear by the root, realizing that the I is empty. Who is getting worried? I am? Where is this I? Can we find it? But this must not just be an intellectual exercise; we must also have a direct experience in our mind, body, and energy, else it has no hold. We must have this experience of no I to its fullest due to our habitual pattern of building everything around the human I, me, you, whether consciously or unconsciously. If we have an unstable experience of not finding the I, we get confused and it will only unbalance us even more so. Therefore Mikao Usui placed very specific practices within his teachings to provide a solid direct experience of emptiness, to help us let go of clinging to our worry, clinging to the I.

In common sense, there are two ways to understand something: as a subject and as an object. A subject exists first and makes it possible for an object to exist. "I" as my subject always comes first, and then I can recognize an object as mine or yours... We don't know what the "I" is, so finally the "I" disappears. If the subject disappears, very naturally its object disappears. Finally silence – there's nothing to say.
– The Light That Shines Through Infinity by Dainin Katagiri

Be grateful. Most of the time we are not being grateful due to being angry and worried. Anger is often related to the past and worry is often related to the future, while being grateful is linked to the present moment. We are not being grateful for the present moment, labelling the present moment as good or bad, as this or that, always being dualistic. Hence being grateful also is about emptiness and non-duality. Thus we also can say that the first three precepts are about letting go of the three times of past, present, future. When we are in that state of mind of emptiness, we have also let go of these three times and thus we are free from anger and worry. Free from anger and worry, we can be grateful for all that is, no matter what may happen.

As long as you are involved in dualistic concepts, it is not possible for you to observe our precepts. So how to get out of dualistic concepts and fill our being with gratitude is the point of practice.
– Wind Bell: Teachings from the San Francisco Zen Center

Practice diligently. Diligently we need to remember our non-dual empty essence, because due to our habitual pattern we are pulled back again and again into our dual state of mind. Hence again and again we need to rest our mind in our True Self. But to do this we first have to know what our True Self is, else how can we remember it again and again? And even if we have had our first direct experience, maybe through reiju, we still might not be able to remember it again because our habitual patterns are too strong. This, again, is why Mikao Usui placed very specific meditation practices within his teachings. Practice diligently is therefore twofold: practice the meditation practices diligently and remember our True Self diligently. This is real meditation.

If you don't try to better yourself daily, you will easily be led astray. If you don't cultivate your practice daily, it will rust. So here you must not lose track of your True Self, and [you must]

attain Buddhahood every day. You have to approach your food as if you were attaining Buddhahood. In all situations, never lose sight of the True Self.
– Discovering the True Self by Kōdō Sawaki

Be true to your way and your being. We can only really be true to our way and our being if we have let go of our anger and worry. Thus we also can see a certain stepladder within this precept. But don't see it too literally: rather than a line with steps we can climb to reach a final destination, it is more round, like a circle. First we soften our anger and worry and then we start to be a bit more grateful which helps us to be more true to our way and our being and therefore we are more compassionate to ourselves and hence we will be more compassionate to others. Then we go back to soften more of our anger and worry and we start the cycle again. In fact, like practice diligently, being true to your way and your being also is twofold.

Being true to our way is changeable; it is our dualistic nature. For example, today we do this or we eat that, because that is what we need to do today or feel like eating today, due to today's circumstances. This means that being true to our way is dependent on circumstances. However, we need to perform these acts in a state of mind of non-duality, of being true to our being. Being true to our being is non-changeable; it is emptiness. Or as the Heart Sutra states, form is emptiness and emptiness is form. Hence this precept is about the union of duality and non-duality. Or in other words, every act we do today, duality, we do from a state of mind of the precepts, non-duality. When we reach this point in our practice something wonderful starts to happen... pure compassion.

Show compassion to yourself and others. Pure compassion can only arise when we are in this state of emptiness! Why? Because if our compassion is entangled with all sorts of strings, entangled in the "I", then this is not true, real, pure compassion.

"I will be kind to this person but not to that one." "I love this group of people but not that other group." This is compassion which changes; real compassion does not change according to circumstances or judgements. Mikao Usui placed compassion last in his precepts not because it is the least important! He did this because first we have to let go of our anger and worry, which helps us to then see that we have to be grateful for everything that comes on our path. We have to be true to our way and our being, finding union between duality and non-duality. And only then can we have real compassion.

Therefore, *show compassion to yourself and others* is in essence about letting go of the "I". When there is no "I", then there is no you, and all we have left is true compassion. This is like the rain and the sun we touched upon when discussing the kanji of Reiki. True compassion does not judge, label or distinguish; it just shines, it just rains down. Thus we can start to see that each element of Mikao Usui's teachings is not a separate element at all; they are all interconnected to point us to universal truth, the ultimate reality.

> *When you see kindness as an object for you to attain, you have to tell yourself: just be kind. But if you go beyond even the thought of being kind, there is no object. If you don't see an object, very naturally there is no subject – your sense of individual self drops off. What's left? Just the state of being completely kind; your life is just the pure activity of kindness itself.*
> *– The Light That Shines Through Infinity by Dainin Katagiri*

All these teachers point out the same thing: emptiness. Hence the whole precept is about emptiness. The precepts are not just a few sentences; they are deep teachings to explain emptiness to us. Thus do not read them mindlessly, as just some words on a piece of paper. Go deeper, go into the deepest layer of the precepts and discover that they are about emptiness, no object –

"I", no subject – "you", just compassion.

Some say that Mikao Usui copied the precepts from someone else, but if we get caught up about that we are missing the whole point, and we are intellectualizing Mikao Usui's teachings. As you can see, these teachings are common to Japanese spiritual practices like Zen and are there to help us to understand emptiness. If we debate about whether the precepts are from this or that person, we are getting caught up with the finger pointing to the moon instead of looking at the moon itself, caught up in talk of the precepts instead of looking at what the precepts themselves are pointing at.

But there is yet another layer to this teaching of Mikao Usui. Whenever we practice any of the meditation practices in the system of Reiki, we have to do it from the place of compassion to ourselves and others; this is our motivation. What does this mean? It means that when we sit down to practice, no matter if it is hands on/off healing on ourselves or jōshin kokyū hō or any of the other methods, we start with the mindset that we do this to remember our own inner great bright light, our emptiness, for the sake of others. For the sake of others means that we want to help others to also remember their great bright light. This is the deepest level of compassion we can have for ourselves and others.

In other words, our sitting must be based on the compassionate desire to save all sentient beings by means of calming the mind.
– Introduction to Zen Training: A Physical Approach to Meditation and Mind-Body Training by Omori Sogen

Morning and evening perform gassho. Now Mikao Usui gives us some very important instructions on how to practice. Every morning and evening we have to perform gassho. Gassho is bringing our hands together in prayer position, left hand and right hand in union. Thus gassho stands for non-duality, the union of left and right, this and that, here and there. Plus he instructs us to practice at least twice a day. There is no specific amount of time we have to practice. In some Reiki schools they say recite the precepts three times. But in reality we all know that reciting them three times will not suddenly mean we have no more anger and worry. Three times is the bare minimum. In fact we might need to chant the precepts 45 minutes in the morning and 45 minutes in the evening so that we can gain control over our monkey mind. But there is another layer to this: perform gassho represents the body aspect. Mikao Usui is pointing out that we have to use our body in the right way, in the right position, when we perform any of the practices within his teachings, as the body is the vehicle for our mind and energy!

In Buddhism, the left side is a symbol of auspiciousness and supreme happiness; the right side is a symbol of dynamic, creative life. On the left, the opportunity of auspiciousness is always open to everybody... On the right, you accept any aspect of human life, stand up, and live in a positive way.
– The Light That Shines Through Infinity by Dainin Katagiri

Keep in your mind: Here Mikao Usui instructs us that when we are sitting in gassho and we are chanting, we have to keep the precepts in our mind. This means, do not chant mindlessly: focus. Maybe we know the precepts by heart and then when we chant we are just chanting by rote and not focused at all. If we chant that way, we do not gain control over our confused distracted mind and therefore we will never lay bare our innate emptiness. But this teaching is not just for when we chant the precepts; it is also about when we perform hands on/off healing and any of the other practices within the system of Reiki. We must keep our mind focused. We will discuss this later as it is one of the more important elements. And at the deepest level, we have to keep the essence of the precepts in our mind, emptiness, in all we do. This is the most important of all. But we cannot just think that we are empty, which would be like wishing a teacup full of tea to be empty. We have to apply a method first, to find that emptiness.

Chant with your mouth. Here Mikao Usui is telling us to chant the precepts with our mouth, thus out loud, and not silently in our mind. Chanting is an important element in many Japanese spiritual practices. Why? Because it is the link between our body and mind. The body is very tangible and the mind is very subtle. And chanting is just in between; thus it is the link between body and mind. And again, if we really think about it, then chanting the precepts once or twice or three times is not enough to stimulate our inner energy and free it up of all our stuck emotions and trauma. We need to chant again and again and again. In fact we need to chant until we have embodied the precepts in all we do during the day, and even then we need to keep going.

Improve your mind-body. Here is yet another very important element to the puzzle of Mikao Usui's teachings which many teachers often do not talk about: shinshin kaizen, improve your mind-body. It is so important that there is a whole chapter dedicated to this aspect of the precepts. But for now it will suffice to say that this again is a very common viewpoint within Japanese spiritual practices like Zen, for example. It is about harmonizing our mind and body, which normally are not in harmony at all. And thus we get angry and worried. Plus, and this is another important element, it points to our body. We have to go within our body because that is the vehicle for our mind at this moment in time. Thus we have to be centered within our body and not airy fairy, out of our body.

Body and mind working as one is perfected in a moment. If it continues for one's whole life, it is Buddha.
– Discovering the True Self by Kōdō Sawaki

Here we have looked at the precepts in a nutshell. But there are many layers to the precepts and how they relate to the system of

Reiki. Thus we will come back to the precepts again and again to help gain a deeper understanding as to why Mikao Usui put them within his teachings and how important they are to our direct experience, how important it is that we embody the precepts in our daily life.

Many people think that the system of Reiki is about some magical symbols and mantras. and that once attuned or initiated, a Reiki practitioner then can do some magical spells for healing. But in fact the system of Reiki is all about the embodiment of the precepts in all we do during our day, for today. This is the real spiritual blessing and this is also a manifestation of the deepest healing we can lay bare – emptiness – non-duality – this is the spiritual medicine of 10.000 illnesses.

For the members of our association, please keep this in mind that the more you have a higher virtue in yourself the stronger your spiritual energy becomes.

– Reiki Ryôhô no Shiori, handed out by the Usui Reiki Ryôhô Gakkai

Even the Usui Reiki Ryôhô Gakkai (Usui Reiki Healing Method Learning Society, founded in Japan in the 1920s) points out that through the embodiment of the precepts, virtues, the stronger our spiritual energy becomes. And this is why the precepts are the foundation of the system of Reiki. Why? Because anger, worry, jealousy, greed – you name it – eat up our energy. Embodying the precepts in all we do, replenishes and feeds that energy, and makes it stronger.

Your understanding of precepts is not a matter of intellectual teaching; it is a matter of direct experience. The universe is going in a certain system and rhythm. It's not random. When that rhythm is alive in human life, it is called the precepts.

– The Light That Shines Through Infinity by Dainin Katagiri

Chapter 5:

Mind Body Speech

Mind, Body, Speech are very important elements within traditional Japanese spiritual practices and teachings and we can see them clearly portrayed within the system of Reiki. We first become aware of them in the kanji of Reiki, with the three mouths and of course we see them very clearly within the precepts. Remember…

> Morning and evening perform gassho – **body**
> Keep in your mind – **mind**
> Chant with your mouth – **speech/energy/breath**

Here we can see a clear reference to mind, body, speech, or as it is called in Japan, sanmitsu – the three mysteries. First we have to harmonize these three mysteries of mind, body, speech within our own being and when that starts to happen we slowly harmonize with the three mysteries of the universe. This harmony in turn will lay bare our non-dual nature.

Because Reiki Therapy improves self-healing ability by using the spiritual energy coming from your own body, it's safe and anyone can do it.
– September 1974, Usui Reiki Therapy Association Headquarters Chairman Toyokazu Kazuwa (Reiki Ryôhô no Shiori booklet, handed out by the Usui Reiki Ryôhô Gakkai)

Let's start with the body. The body is the vehicle for our mind and energy. Speech is also energy and breath; they are in essence one and the same. Body, mind, and energy are interlinked; for example, to calm our mind we need first to adjust our body and energy. Our mind depends on our energy and our energy depends on our physical body. Our physical body is also sustained by our energy and the quality of our mind. We all know that when we are angry, our body becomes contracted and therefore our energy cannot flow through our body in a free flowing way.

For most of his students, Mikao Usui started with a focus on the body; he did this because it is the easiest way to start. This is also seen within Yoga or Tai Chi, for example, in which you first start with your body. Our body is the most tangible of the three mysteries, mind the most subtle and energy is in between. Hence energy/breath/speech is the link between the body and mind.

The body comes out of the Way and what is derived from the Way is also the body. Correcting one's posture is the same thing as learning the Way by means of the body, that is, turning the whole universe into one's own body.
− Introduction to Zen Training: A Physical Approach to Meditation and Mind-Body Training by Omori Sogen

So first Mikao Usui taught hands on healing: touching our body, becoming aware of our physicality and making friends with our own body. When we place the hands on our own body we not only start to soften the tissues, but if our mind stays open we also touch upon the energy within our physical body. But if we touch our own body while we are slumped over or while our mind is distracted, then the energy will not flow smoothly through our body and therefore our hands on healing practice will lose its full potential.

This is the same with the other practices within the system of Reiki. When we chant the precepts or chant the mantras of Okuden Reiki II and Shinpiden Reiki III, or when we do the meditation practices, we first of all have to place our body in the right position, a stable position. The more stable the position is, upright, not too tense and not too loose, just like a guitar string is neither too loose nor too tight, the more our energy will flow through the energy channels in a straight and effective way. And with a stable body position, the more stable our mind becomes. This is why, if we look closely, a correct meditation posture is like a triangle: the base is solid and wide, and the top is focused.

The breath is a link between our body and mind, a way to anchor our mind in the body so that we can realize the wide open nature of our mind. If we are not anchored, our mind will go all over the place, just like a balloon taken by the wind here, there and everywhere. Anchoring means that we tie a solid object to the string of the balloon, the balloon can still move but it is not taken here, there and everywhere; the monkey mind is under control. This is why we find very specific breathing and chanting practices within the system of Reiki and we do these practices to gain control over our energy, which ultimately helps to have the direct realization of our True Self.

Breath is the bridge which connects life to consciousness, which unites your body to your thoughts.
– Thich Nhat Hanh

It is through the mind that we experience this great bright light, compassion and wisdom, and this is why we see that Mikao Usui points towards the mind again and again. The precepts, for example, are all about the mind. Many people think that the system of Reiki is an energetic practice but they forget the body and mind aspect, and if we look carefully, we can see that energy follows the mind. If we think of Reiki only as an energy practice, then our practice is like a boat without a steering wheel and sails; we go from here to there and will never reach our destination, illumination. Mind, body, energy need to be in complete harmony with each other and if we leave any of these practices out, the whole practice loses its essence. This is why we have to anchor the mind in the body, in the hara.

If the body is corrected, mind and breath will be reasonably correct in themselves. It is no use correcting mind and respiration when the body is neglected and the posture incorrect.
– Introduction to Zen Training: A Physical Approach to Meditation and Mind-Body Training by Omori Sogen

Sanmitsu – mind, body, speech – also represents visualization = mind, mudra = body, and chanting = speech. We can clearly see these aspects within Mikao Usui's teachings. We visualize the breath moving during the meditation practices and we visualize the symbols. At the deepest level, mind is the state of mind of emptiness. Mudras often are seen just as specific hand movements, but mudra is also how we use our whole physical body. We can find this in hands on/off healing and of course how we sit during the meditation practices or how we stand when we perform reiju. At the deepest level, mudra is how we sit, walk, sleep, and more; it is how we use our body. Chanting is the speech element; we see this in chanting the precepts and chanting the mantras within the system of Reiki. At the deepest level, speech is not just chanting, but is every word which comes out of our mouth.

Instructing us through the precepts, Mikao Usui tells us that to truly benefit from his teachings and to have this direct experience of our True Self, we need to include mind, body, speech in all of the practice: within hands on/off healing, within the meditation practices like jōshin kokyū hō, within the mantras and symbols and within the reiju. In fact, he is pointing out that we need the unification of these three elements in our daily life, in all we do. To give a small example of what happens if our mind, body, and speech/energy are not in harmony, if we perform hands on healing on ourselves and our mind is all over the place, not focused, then our energy also is all over the place and not focused. This in turn means that we are not creating the right environment for true healing to take place. We are not applying the method to its fullest, the cake we are making might not be satisfying because we left out one ingredient. Our house might not be stable because we missed a wall or a roof. We need this right environment to stimulate the inner fire, the mist, and the raining down as we saw within the kanji of Reiki. These inner workings are necessary for laying bare the ultimate layer of emptiness, buddha nature, our True Self.

When mind moves, ki moves.
– Yuasa Yasuo, The Body, Self-Cultivation, and Ki-Energy

Chapter 6:

Improve Mind-Body

Within the precepts we also find the Japanese sentence *shinshin kaizen* 心身改善 which is yet another important teaching and pointer that Mikao Usui left us.

Shinshin 心身 mind-body
Kaizen 改善 improve

The fact that Mikao Usui included *shinshin kaizen* within his precepts shows that he must have found it an important element. In fact, he used it as the closing thought to these instructions, an essential part of the precepts for the students of Mikao Usui's times and for us in our times.

But what does *shinshin kaizen* – improve mind-body – really mean?

From a traditional Japanese perspective it means the unification of our mind-body, as normally our mind and body are not in harmony. This unification really only takes place when we improve ourselves, when we practice the meditation practices Mikao Usui put in his system. Practicing the system of Reiki is a lifelong practice, improvement upon improvement, to move us toward this unification, this harmony.

Simply said, we can see that the body is right here; it is not distracted by the past, present, or future. Or in other words, our physical body is not in the past, neither is it in the future and neither is it contemplating the present moment. Our body is essentially free of these three times. But our mind is always distracted by the past, present, and future. And therefore there is a gap between our mind and our body: there is no harmony or unity.

This approach to body and mind as a unity was not generally viewed as a "naturally" experienced phenomenon, however, but rather as a synergy requiring conscious effort and special training (shugyō 修行). This training often took the form of meditation (either sitting meditation or more dynamic types of meditation through movement), as a practice through which the harmony of mind and body could be cultivated. The goal of such training was typically expressed as the attainment of an "awakening" (satori 悟り).
– Yuasa Yasuo's Theory of the Body by Britta Boutry-Stadelmann

Thus from a traditional Japanese approach, this improvement of mind-body is in essence only truly realized when we attain satori, spiritual awakening. Mikao Usui thus was pointing within his teachings to enlightenment, harmony between mind-body.

So the old Gakkai members said that Usui Sensei taught the way to Satori very intensely to those who had achieved a certain level.
– Hiroshi Doi

This *satori* is again the unity of mind-body, *shinshin kaizen* – the improvement of our mind-body. It also was, according to Hiroshi Doi, the focus of Mikao Usui's teachings, especially to some of his students who had achieved a certain level. And Mikao Usui was teaching the way of satori, improve mind-body, quite intensely. It was not an easy five day course but an intense lifelong practice/improvement.

Usui Sensei did not give additional healing trainings but I heard that he often taught classes about a Shihan's mental attitude in order to improve one's teaching methods when teaching about healing to the members. Though his one-on-one Shinpi-den lecture did not include healing training, I also heard that Usui Sensei's mentorship greatly enhanced the healing ability of many of the Shinpi-den practitioners, as it strengthened their resonance with the Universe and encouraged the awareness that a human is the small universe derived from the Great Universe.

– Hiroshi Doi

Here Hiroshi Doi points out something very important and something that often is overlooked in many modern teachings of the system of Reiki. Doi points out that Mikao Usui was not teaching additional healing trainings per se during his one-on-one Shinpiden teachings, but whatever he was teaching strengthened his students' resonance with the universe. We can almost be certain that Mikao Usui was teaching those students specific meditation practices, *shugyō* 修行, to improve their mind-body. And through this improvement of mind-body – *shinshin kaizen* – their healing ability was greatly enhanced! Satori also stands for understanding; hence when we have this direct experience of satori we start to understand the mysteries of life. This is also why Mikao Usui called his Reiki level III Shinpiden, as Shinpiden stands for mystery teachings, the mystery of life. But we only start to understand this through these specific practices and teachings and then, as we continue our practice, we understand that everything is emptiness. This becomes more apparent when we take a closer look at the whole structure of Mikao Usui's teachings.

We also can see that by placing *shinshin kaizen* within the precepts, Mikao Usui based his teachings on the teachers of old, who also had this direct experience of satori.

For example, Eisai (1141-1215), founder of Rinzai Zen, called this realization of mind-body *shinshin ichinyo* 心身一如, mind-body oneness.

And Dōgen (1200-1253), founder of Sōtō Zen, called this realization *shinjin datsuraku* 身心脱落, the dropping-off of body-mind. This concept of dropping body-mind means dropping the distinction between body and mind.

And Myōe (明恵 1173-1232) called this realization *shinjin*

gyōnen 心身凝然, unshakable mind-body.

Thus by looking at teachers like Dōgen, teachers of old, we start to see what and how Mikao Usui was trying to teach: *shinshin kaizen*, perfect harmony between mind and body.

This of course is not an easy task. This is why Mikao Usui instructed us to meditate and recite the precepts on a daily basis, so that one day we might have the direct full experience of mind-body harmony. And this is why we do just that – continue our daily meditations, recitations, and practices to strengthen and encourage, as Hiroshi Doi said, our resonance with the Universe and our awareness that we ourselves are "a small universe derived from the Great Universe."

The Way of learning with the mind also is included in the realm of physical realization and must be interrelated to the body and expressed through our physical activities. Otherwise, it cannot be regarded as the true Way of learning with the mind.
– Introduction to Zen Training: A Physical Approach to Meditation and Mind-Body Training by Omori Sogen

Thus when we have that direct experience of the mind of emptiness – non-duality – we have to express this in our daily dual activities, our interactions with others. We integrate the experience by helping others, by being compassionate to others. This is also why compassion for others is such an important element, as it involves both our mind and our body! The daily activity of compassion is expressed from our direct experience of the precepts, of emptiness, non-duality.

To really understand the meaning of life, we have to go beyond thinking and experience the vast scale of life directly, with our own body and mind.
– The Light That Shines Through Infinity by Dainin Katagiri

Chapter 7:

Great Bright Light

Usui Sensei taught Shinpiden students one on one and he showed them the kanji dai kômyô, which indicated the consciousness of a Shinpiden practitioner.
– Hiroshi Doi, Spain 2015 seminar

As we have seen, the precepts are a description of the great bright light 大光明 dai kômyô, of emptiness, non-duality. This means that when we start to practice the system of Reiki we need to be pointed towards this great bright light, not later, but right at the beginning at Shoden Reiki I. Why? Imagine I want to go and visit a friend in Paris. To do this I need to have their address in Paris, I need to know where to go, else I will not reach my destination. Therefore we need to know straight away at the beginning why we practice and what our destination is, else we will become lost.

This also means that by knowing my destination I can create a straight path towards the destination. None of us knows when our time to die will come, so better to get straight to our destination of our True Self, because if we die it is too late to practice. And at the moment of death we will have our biggest test ever: can we die without anger and worry, can we die being grateful for everything in our life, can we die being true to our way and our being, and can we die in a compassionate way.

Therefore, it is absolutely necessary for us to be always aware of our True Selves twenty-four hours a day, without deviation.
– Introduction to Zen Training: A Physical Approach to Meditation and Mind-Body Training by Omori Sogen

Knowing this non-dual destination, we also need to nurture our non-dual True Self again and again, else we fall into the trap of duality over and over. What does that mean? That whatever we practice, we need to see it from a non-dual perspective. Of course we all live in a dual world and we should not ignore this, but we can live in this dual world with a state of mind of non-duality. Because it is only in that state of mind that we can truly lead a peaceful life and have a peaceful world.

Thus if in our practice and teachings, we keep saying things like, "This is a higher vibration than that," "This a different kind of Reiki than that," "I need to connect to your energy," "I am more evolved than you because I am a Reiki Master," then we are promoting duality and we will not be able to lay bare our non-dual nature. This would be like having the address of my friend in Paris but now I am taking the train to Copenhagen; I will not reach my destination. I know that now people may say, "But hey, we just have a little side trip to Copenhagen." But when you are in Copenhagen you get caught up by Copenhagen and you forget your real destination. And again, who knows when we will die? Maybe we die in Copenhagen and therefore we have never rediscovered our True Self. Why take a detour if you can go straight to the core of the teachings?!

The Great Light has no colour, yet it is all colours. It transcends past, present and future. It existed before the universe appeared and it will exist after the universe is gone. And although this Great Light can be talked about for eons, it cannot be explained in words. Nor can it be seen with the most precise microscope or the most powerful telescope. It is simply magnificent beyond description, and it can be seen only with Wisdom's Eye... Our basic nature is clearer than the sky and is no different from Buddha.
– Ven. Tong Songchol

Thus Mikao Usui pointed straight from the beginning of his

teachings towards this great bright light, this non-dual nature. We not only see this within the precepts as they are about non-duality, but we also know that he performed reiju on his students. Reiju is a remembering of who we are: a great bright light. Thus by performing reiju, Mikao Usui was showing his students the destination, their inner luminosity. It is like he put his students on the path, right at the start, the path of self-illumination. But the student has to walk this path themselves of course; no one else can do this.

Here is another example: take a bow and arrow. If I want to hit a specific target I need to aim at the target. If I want to hit that tree over there, I do not aim at the rock; I aim at the tree. But now we have to do something; we have to let go of the arrow, else it will never hit the target. So we know the target and now we need to let go, else we will be distracted by the target itself. This means we just need to practice without the idea of a goal. And yet we have to aim again and again and we have to let go again and again. Why do we have to aim again and again? Because we often get sidetracked and we lose sight of our destination, lose our aim! But each time we reaffirm our aim we also then have to let go. This is the way to practice. We will come back to this letting go later as it is a very important concept for when we practice the five elements within the system of Reiki.

This is why it is of utmost importance that we know why we are practicing, what our aim is, and how to lay bare what we are aiming at. And this is why it is important to start straight away, when we first enter the path of the system of Reiki, to focus on non-duality, emptiness, and inner illumination. If we start this later within our practice it will be more difficult to find the way to our inner light. It will be like moving into a house of non-attachment, to start gathering all sorts of objects that we become attached to, and then later to learn that we have to let these objects go. This will be difficult if over time we have become so attached to these wonderful shiny objects we have gathered. Thus is it better not to collect all sorts of lovely objects in our practice but instead to begin with a clear vision and understanding of what is at the heart of our practice. If we do this, as we progress in our practice it will be much easier to let go if we have become attached to fewer things along the way. The bag of our practice can be as full or as empty as we make it, on our way to the destination of emptiness, of non-duality. But empty is always easier.

The Natural Law of the Great Universe and each human spirit as a small universe must be constantly united and exist as One.
– note from a student of Mikao Usui

Chapter 8:

Hara – Our Center

Before we look at how to practice and all the different practices within the system of Reiki, we have to examine one more important element that Mikao Usui pointed out: the hara. Both Mikao Usui and Mrs. Takata, who brought the system of Reiki to the West, pointed out the hara many times in their words and teachings. They did this because the hara is central to the practice, in more ways than one.

Excerpt from Mrs. Takata's diary, December 10th, 1935:
Meaning of "Reiki" Energy within oneself, when concentrated and applied to patient, will cure all ailments – it is nature's greatest cure, which requires no drugs. It helps in all respects, human and animal life. In order to concentrate, one must purify one's thoughts in words and in thoughts and to meditate to let the "energy" come out from within. It lies in the bottom of the stomach about 2 inches below the navel. Sit in a comfortable position, close your eyes, concentrate on your thoughts and relax...

The hara is an energy center, focus point, at the bottom of your stomach, approximately two inches below your navel. It is one of the essential elements within most Japanese spiritual practices.

The Japanese feel that hara can help not only your everyday life, but that it can be a way to attain the ultimate enlightenment.
– The Art and the Way of Hara by Seigen Yamaoka

As we have seen, Mikao Usui's teachings aimed to help his students realize ultimate enlightenment. Therefore, like many Japanese spiritual teachers, he also used the hara within his system.

The Japanese word hara 腹 has many meanings: abdomen, mind, courage, one's true intention or motive, center, true center of a person, the proper seat of the mind, true mind. And in the Japanese culture, there are some wonderful sentences which describe the different meanings of hara:

Hara ga tatsu – to be angry
Hara wo waru – a heart to heart talk
Hara ga dekite iru – having a calm mind even in times of emergency
Hara ga chii-sai – narrow-minded
Hara ga suwaru – to be mentally stable and unshakable
Hara o kimeru – to make one's mind up
Hara ga futoi – to be courageous – a large heart

So as we can see, the word hara means not just abdomen, not just the physical center of the body, but much, much more. This is why it is such an integral part of Mikao Usui's teachings.

Let's look at the precepts, and see how the hara fits in:

Do not anger
Do not worry
Be grateful
Be true to your way and your being
Show compassion to yourself and others

First of all, to practice the system of Reiki we need to make up our mind to start to practice: *hara o kimeru*. We have to have a very clear intention to practice, else we never will walk the path. Then we need to slowly let go of our anger, so that we will find composure and not be angry all the time: *hara ga tatsu*. Then we start to let go of our worry and we become calm in all situations: *hara ga dekite iru*. To be grateful, we need to open our mind and find tolerance, so we have to let go of our narrow-mindedness: *hara ga chii-sai*. When we are true to our way and our being, we need to be mentally stable: *hara ga suwaru*. And to show compassion to ourselves and others, we need to have a large heart: *hara ga futoi*.

Thus hidden deep within the precepts, we find the concept of hara. And the more we embody the precepts in our daily life, the more we become *a person of hara*, a person who embodies stability in their daily life.

The general description of a person of hara is someone with courage, will power, strength, determination, character, integrity, honesty, and patience. Such a person is also known as a person with a "big hara". That is, they are generous, compassionate, and understanding.

– The Art and the Way of Hara by Seigen Yamaoka

Doesn't what Seigen Yamaoka describe in this quote represent a person who has embodied the precepts? Of course. We can see the concept of hara clearly within the precepts; we just have to look. And then we have to look again. Often we only look at the words, the surface teaching, in the precepts. But there are many hidden words, inner teachings, to be found there. And to see these inner teachings we have to dig deeper; we have to practice and look beyond the initial meaning.

When we look at the meditation practices taught within Japanese Reiki traditions, we see a practice called jōshin kokyū hō. This practice focuses on the hara, breathing deeply into the hara so that the practitioner can become more stable and centered. But for this meditation to really have any benefit, we have to keep doing it again and again and again so that we can rediscover our hara, our center.

It takes time, concentration, patience and endurance to meditate.

Many give up before achieving any results. Because this practice is so relaxing, we may stop at this point in the meditative process and do it only for the purpose of relaxation. But you must persist in order to be introduced to the hara.
– *The Art and the Way of Hara by Seigen Yamaoka*

This is what many teachers teach now as the system of Reiki: a relaxation practice, a way to relieve stress. But that doesn't do Mikao Usui any honor at all, because his teachings are so much more than relaxation. If we want to relax, we might just as well have a massage or a nap. Mikao Usui's teachings, if practiced in the right way, are a way to remember and experience our True Self.

When we look at the mantras taught within the system of Reiki, we also can see the hara there. In order to chant mantras correctly from a Japanese spiritual perspective, we need to chant them from the hara. This deep kind of chanting creates a resonance which moves through our whole being from our center, our hara. Through prolonged chanting in this way, we can embody the precepts more and more in our daily life, so that again we can become a person of hara.

Since we chant these words with energy from the abdomen, it naturally creates the repetition of deep breathing from the belly... Through this breathing, the power in the physical body is increased.
– *The Essence of Shinto: Japan's Spiritual Heart by Motohisa Yamakage*

This deep kind of chanting from the hara is used in all major Japanese spiritual teachings, from Shinto to Shugendo to Tendai Buddhism, and to Mikao Usui's teachings. The main purpose of this deep hara chanting, in all teachings, is that we may remember our True Self. It is to create the right environment for the fire, the mist and the rain, as is pointed out within the kanji of Reiki. When we look at the symbols within the system of Reiki, we can see the hara in there as well. For example, the first symbol, when visualized, goes inwards. Why does it go inward? By going inward, we are able to rediscover our hara, our center, so that we can become centered in our daily life. In doing this, going inward to our center, we slowly start to embody the symbol, embody its meaning. Traditionally you would use the symbols for internal meditations to rediscover your True Self. For this, the True Self, is the center of the universal flow of divine consciousness.

In other words, we must never allow ourselves to forget the concept of chushin, our center. All things are controlled by the stability and the quality of their center, the place where their being is born. We may call this place the life force, or kannagara, the universal flow of divine consciousness. Whatever you wish to call it, it is the force that comes from our hara.

– a teaching from Morihei Ueshiba, founder of Aikido, from the book Principles of Aikido by Mitsugi Saotome

But here comes the interesting part... the physical aspect of the hara is just a signpost; in the deeper levels of our practice we also need to let go of the hara. Takuan Soho, a famous Zen master (1573-1645), taught that focusing on the hara applies to a person under training but that a person who goes deep into their personal practice lets go of resting their mind on the hara. Thus the focus on our hara is merely a stepping stone! But we don't throw away the stepping stone too quickly else we sink; we sink into the sea of anger and worry, of not being grateful, not being true to our way and our being, and not being compassionate to ourselves and others. If we throw our stepping stones away too soon, we have a house without a solid foundation. And when we go deeper into our practice, the house might collapse and we would have to start again, which would be a pity after all the practice we have done. So be careful... check in with a good, qualified teacher who knows about the hara through their own personal dedicated practice before you throw away the stepping stone of physically focusing on the hara during your meditations.

The final point to be made about meditation is that although hara plays an important part, you can become attached to it, in which case hara becomes a crutch and a hindrance. In final analysis, you must become free even of hara.

– The Art and the Way of Hara by Seigen Yamaoka

Due to modernization in Japan, as in most countries, we see that lots of teachings are losing this ancient hara practice and focus. But even as we live in a modern time, we still can pick up these old tried and true teachings which already have brought so much benefit to many people around the world. This is why even within some Japanese teachings of the system of Reiki we find no mention of the hara, or we might not even find teachings like sanmitsu – mind, body, speech – which Mikao Usui pointed out so clearly within the precepts. In some cases it seems like it has been completely overlooked, even by Japanese Reiki teachers.

One of the major casualties of the Japanese language's rapid and ongoing evolution is the diminishing use of body-related phrases – a phenomenon that reflects how Japanese people's once-visceral connection between their bodies and minds is these days rapidly attenuating.

– The Japan Times (oldest English daily newspaper in Japan)

Thus, if we want to get the desired result of remembering our True Self, it is important to include the ancient Japanese practice of hara as Mikao Usui pointed out within his teachings, so that we each can become a person of hara and embody the precepts in our daily life. For it is through this personal practice, an embodiment of hara, that the world can become a better place, a place of healing and compassion.

The mere fact that these words are frequently used in Japanese society should not be taken to indicate that all citizens of modern Japan possess a deep or innate understanding of ki and hara.
– *The Japanese Way of the Artist by H.E. Davey*

Chapter 9:

Practice Tips

Now that we have looked at the foundation of the system of Reiki, we can look at how to practice. Let's explore this a bit, as practicing in the right way is an important element. We want to create the right environment in which we have the fire, the steam and the rain, a natural environment within ourselves. We could say practice makes perfect, but that is not true; if we practice in the wrong way, we get the wrong result or no result at all. Again, if we make a cake and we mix the ingredients in the wrong way, then our cake might not even be edible. Or if we haven't made a solid foundation of a house, we might put the roof on top and the whole house collapses. Hence it is better to say, as one teacher of mine pointed out once, perfect practice makes perfect. Mikao Usui pointed out how to practice perfectly within the word Reiki, within the precepts, and with 大光明 dai kômyô.

> *"Everlasting light" is constantly illuminating your life, but the stubborn human consciousness cannot believe it. So first we have to open ourselves to accept that light. Everyone always forgets this first practice.*
> *– The Light That Shines Through Infinity by Dainin Katagiri*

Thus no matter if we practice any of the five elements within the system of Reiki, we have to start with the right attitude and motivation as Mikao Usui taught us. Just to recap, the five elements are these: the precepts, meditation practices, hands on/off healing, symbols and mantras, and the reiju. And when we practice any of these or all of them together, we need to infuse our practice with the essence of Reiki, the essence of the system of Reiki.

First we check our body, breath, mind.

Put your body in the right posture; check if you are too tight or if you are too loose. It is fine to sit in a chair if you can't sit on a pillow in a traditional meditation position. But when you sit on a chair, make sure you have your feet flat on the ground and you do not lean back against the back of the chair. This way you start to sit up straight, which is what you want to do, as it helps your breathing.

Now check your breathing. Are you breathing high up in your chest or are you breathing deep down into your belly? We have to make sure, in a gentle way without forcing anything, that we breathe deep into the hara. The top of the body stays stationary, not too tight, not too loose, while the belly region moves out on the inhale and in on the exhale. This way the belly, the hara, becomes the bellows to ignite the inner fire that is needed to create the right environment for our practice.

Now check your mind. We always do it in this order; why? Because when our body posture is correct, our breathing falls much more easily into the hara, and this in turn will help us to calm our mind. So what do we have to check in our mind? First we check if we are agitated or not; if you are agitated or distracted, try in a gentle way to calm your mind. If that doesn't work, just focus on your body and breathing. Then we have to aim ourselves toward our target: the direct experience of emptiness, of our True Self. Now let go. Don't force it. Just sit, breathe, focus, aim, and then let go.

If we aim in our practice just at healing the pain in our knee, or we aim just at feeling relaxed, or falling asleep, or if we do not aim at all, then we will never hit our target, our True Self, the direct experience of emptiness, non-duality. Thus each time check what your target is; be very clear about it. This in turn also helps with your motivation; why do you practice the system of Reiki? The clearer the target the easier it is for the arrow to hit the mark: bullseye, right into the eye of your True Self.

Now mix into this the motivation we have found within the precepts: compassion. We practice to be compassionate to ourselves and we also do this for the sake of others. In other words, we practice for ourselves so that we have the direct experience of our great bright light so that we can help others to find their great bright light. That is really our motivation. When we have this kind of motivation, our practice becomes much more juicy; it is not a dry practice anymore. A dry practice is an egocentric practice, just for our own self. But to let it rain onto ourselves and others, we need to have a juicy practice; hence we have compassion for others in all that we do and we bring this to our practice. Please do not think this is just a simple instruction; explore it for yourself and you will find out that this really starts to change your practice. All the masters of old pointed this out as well.

Next mix in emptiness – non-duality – this will amplify the compassion to yourself and others. But this is not an easy step. First we can start with the intellectual understanding of it, that we are all interconnected. You are everything and everything is you. But if we still have a lot of worry, for example, then this step is not right for us at the moment, as it might even trigger more fear and worry. Then we just wait, continuing our practice, until our foundation, our base, our hara is more stable. Later on, through practicing again and again, we might slowly start to have glimpses of this emptiness within our own mind, body, speech. But until then, we first set our mind towards this understanding so that we can practice correctly. Again do not force this; we cannot make something empty by just wishing it to be empty.

As for the images and sounds which arise during meditation, they are all right if they do not give rise to dualistic thought and if they do not cause thoughts to follow.

—Introduction to Zen Training: A Physical Approach to Meditation and Mind-Body Training by Omori Sogen

Mixing emptiness into the practice is also important as it helps us not to get distracted by what we may experience during the practices. Whatever thoughts arise, let them come and straight away let them go. Do not follow these thoughts as it will only give rise to duality and that is not what any of the practices are about. For that we need no practice; we have already enough dualistic thoughts.

And now we practice any of the five elements of the system of Reiki. But hang on, there is more...

While we are practicing we have to make sure that our mind, especially our mind, stays in the right posture, stays in emptiness so to speak. But as we have not had the direct experience of emptiness yet, we have to make sure our mind stays focused, as energy follows the mind. So each time we have to become aware if our mind is straying into the past or future, or analyzing the present moment. When we feel this happening, we bring the mind, gently, back to the practice. No critique, no judgement; just gently bring the mind back. If you practice hands on/off healing for example, bring your mind back to the hands. Through this constant, not too tight, focus, just like a guitar string, we start to be carried away less and less by the past, present and future so that our mind is at rest. And when our mind is at rest we start to have glimpses of our True Self, of emptiness.

This is how we practice in the right way, this is how we create the right environment for spiritual maturation to take place, for that self-illumination to emerge. Through doing this, we can slowly begin to bear the precepts in our mind in all we do during the day. And remember a day consists also of sleeping. Thus when we can remain in the state of mind of the precepts during our waking hours, we slowly start to remain in that state of mind during our sleep as well. Now, when we reach this point, we are kind of practicing day and night. We are not carried away by the daily emotions and by the nightly dreams; we realize that whatever takes place is a manifestation of emptiness. This is really what Mikao Usui pointed out, because it is only through this emptiness and compassion that we start to behave in a humane way, and in expression of the precepts. And through this expression of the precepts in all we do, we create a better world. But this better world, this heaven on earth, first starts with ourselves.

Whatever practice you do – Buddhist practice, Christian practice, or nonreligious practice – when you become aware of the magnificent energy of being arising in your body and mind, you feel fully alive. You are boundless and broad, compassionate and kind. This is the guideline for living as a human being.

– The Light That Shines Through Infinity by Dainin Katagiri

Of course this is not all; there is much more to practicing in a perfect way. Remember the mist in the kanji of Ki; this is a very important teaching. This mist means do not get distracted by what we experience during the practice; we cannot hold onto mist, we cannot grasp it. We often get so distracted by what we feel, hear, or sense during the practice that this grasping becomes an obstacle to perfect practice. In fact when we grasp onto these experiences during the practice, we are being distracted by the present moment. And when we are distracted we are not creating the right environment for our practice to mature. No opening takes place because we fill this opening with grasping and "I". I feel this, I see that, I hear such and such. Thus we are in fact enforcing the "I" instead of letting go of it. In Japanese this no distraction is called: just practice. Don't make any constructs, leave everything as it is. In practicing this way we aim very clearly at emptiness, our True Self. And this also triggers a lot of energy flow through our whole being, because our energy is not being wasted on the past, present, future, is not being wasted on grasping. Please remember this; this is a very important element, often overlooked by many practitioners and teachers.

As soon as you see something, you already start to intellectualize it. As soon as you intellectualize something, it is no longer what you saw.
– Shunryu Suzuki

Chapter 10:

Form and No-Form

All the different practices or techniques are called form, tangible things that we do with our breath, our hands, our posture, our speech... but we also have no-form. While maybe not as easy to get our minds around, no-form is just as important as form. So we will discuss this aspect of the teachings to help us to gain even more out of our practice. The bow and arrow we discussed already is a great example, so let's refocus on this. We first practice with the bow and arrow; we learn how to hold them in the proper way, how to pull the string, etc... and then we aim and then we let go.

Working with the bow and arrow are form. And after we have let go, we practice no-form. When we let go, the arrow still flies towards the target, sometimes we hit the bullseye right in the middle, sometimes the arrow misses the target all together. This is why we have to keep practicing with form until we hit the bullseye again and again; we have to pick up the bow and arrow, and aim, again and again. But we also have to keep practicing with no-form as we let the arrow fly and rest in that open state of mind. This open state of mind of no-form is 大光明 dai kômyô: emptiness, non-duality. And as this is pointed out in the beginning of our journey, either through words, teachings, or through direct experience, reiju, we have to work with it, as well as working with form.

If practitioners discard their various practices and seek to dwell only in that without form, they will not succeed. On the other hand, neither will they succeed if they cling to their practices, seeking to dwell in that which has form.

– The Commentary on the Dainichi-kyô, translation found in

Shingon: Japanese Esoteric Buddhism by Taiko Yamasaki

This means that we first of all have to unify form and no-form. If we only work with the practice and never move beyond the practice – for example if we never move beyond the symbols – then we get stuck. But if we only work with no-form – for example, being Reiki – and we never practice with form, we are also stuck.

Being Reiki is being in a state of mind of emptiness, of non-duality, of the great bright light. This is not easy. These days I hear too many people say, "Just be Reiki," and then they just stand there or sit there and think that they are Reiki. This is kind of fooling ourselves. We have to be utterly honest with ourselves and not fool ourselves because then we get completely distracted and think we have "arrived" at a destination in our practice that we may not even really understand.

Okay, let's get back to how to practice with form and no-form in unison. When we sit down to practice any of the five elements of the system of Reiki, as we have seen in the previous chapter, we add emptiness in the mix, right at the beginning, even if it is just an intellectual understanding. We have to start somewhere. Then we do the actual practice: chanting, hands on/off healing, meditating on the symbols, breathing practices, etc... We might do a specific form practice for say 20 minutes, and then after these 20 minutes of form practice, we completely let go. We let the arrow fly, no-form, and just sit in that space that we have laid bare through the form practice. We might now sit, for example, five minutes or ten minutes or two minutes in the no-form state of mind. This depends entirely on how long the arrow continues to fly.

If the arrow lands on the ground, we will notice that we get distracted by past, present, and future, and this indicates that we are not in this no-form state of mind any more, if we were at all. This therefore also indicates that we then have to go back to form, and this is how we mix form and no-form. If the arrow hits the bullseye we will be in that natural state of emptiness, it flows naturally, not contrived in any way at all. That doesn't mean we have no thoughts. It means that when thoughts arise, and they will, they will dissolve all by themselves, because we now have discovered that these thoughts are also emptiness. Just like waves in the sea which come up and dissolve. The waves are not separate from the rest of the sea; they are also the sea.

Practice with form refers to systematic meditative ritual using mudra, mantra, and visualization. Practice without form, however, is an individual's every action, whether in ritual format or not, as a reflection of universal enlightened wisdom. This is the ultimate, esoteric practice, in which every word is mantra, every bodily movement mudra, and every thought a meditation.
– Shingon: Japanese Esoteric Buddhism by Taiko Yamasaki

As we can see, no-form is the ultimate esoteric practice. This is when we have integrated the precepts, emptiness, non-duality, and the great bright light, in every action we are performing in the day, no matter if we are awake or asleep. This is *really* being Reiki. Hence it is not so easy to "just be Reiki". So please check yourself carefully if you are fooling yourself that you are being Reiki. Because then you are not only fooling yourself, but you also are fooling your students. This is why even if we are teachers ourselves, we need to have a teacher who can help point out our mistakes or misconceptions. Then we can correct them and thus we will not deviate from the way – path.

Chapter 11:

The Three Times

In previous chapters I have mentioned the three times of past, present, and future, and we can see very clearly how Mikao Usui also put these teachings within his system. For example, we see them within the precepts, which really are about not getting distracted by past, present, and future.

So in a way it is quite simple, but at the same time it's really difficult. If we think about "do not anger" – well, often we are angry about something that just happened to us (or happened last week or five years ago), so it's in the past. Yet we are still angry about it, and may also be worried about how it could affect us going forward. When we look at "do not worry", it's often about the future. We worry, "Am I still going to have a job?" And nowadays that is not always the case. I have lots of friends who unfortunately have lost their jobs and been made redundant due to the COVID situation. So we worry about the future. Thus the first two precepts, do not anger and do not worry, are about the past and the future.

Nowadays we often hear phrases like "stay in the now" or "stay in the present moment". But I think sometimes people get a little bit confused with that. And ultimately we even have to let go of the present moment as well. We have to let go of the now. Why is that? Let's look at being grateful. Being grateful is really about letting go of the present moment, of the now. It often happens that we're doing something at that moment but we're distracted, because we are analyzing the now too much, or we are analyzing *in* the now too much. When we think about the past and the future, it is in that present moment. We're not thinking about the past in the past, and we're not thinking about the future in the future. It is in that moment that we are analyzing, ruminating, and therefore we are not grateful for the moment. This is why we need to let go of that moment, because how long is the moment, actually? Is the moment five minutes, or one second, or is the moment two milliseconds? We cannot find that moment because we are already in the next moment. So we want each moment to be left wide open, not to cling to it, not being distracted and over-analyzing. This is emptiness.

The moment you totally let go, uninvolved in either past, present or future, that is only buddha nature by itself.
– As It Is by Tulku Urgyen

However, this is also one of the hardest parts of our practice. Because we can understand not getting distracted by the past; if I carry the past with me all the time I become very heavy with discomfort. I can carry something that is light – look, here I have something very light, a feather, and I put that in my hand. It is very light but if I keep carrying it for one day, or if I keep my hand in this position for one year, man, that becomes really, really heavy! The longer we carry it, the heavier it becomes. Therefore we know when we carry the past, we can understand that we need to let the past go. We also can understand letting go of the future, as the future is always uncertain. We thought we were going to have a great 2020 and 2021: "I'm gonna go on holiday and I'm going to teach all around the world!" Suddenly that fell away. So we know that the future is very uncertain; we don't know the future. We can worry about it but it might never happen!

The Dalai Lama has a really wonderful quote that goes something like this – if you worry about something and you can fix it, then fix it and stop worrying about it. If you worry about something and you can't fix it then what is the use of worrying about it! So stop worrying about it and let it go. We can easily understand these elements about the past and future. But actually being 100% in that present moment is not so easy. We actually have to let go of that moment; we have to be wide open and then we can really enjoy life to its fullest. Most of the time we're not enjoying life to its fullest, either thinking about the past or the future. And often we are contemplating the present moment way too much, we are too much in our heads. For example when I sit in meditation and I think, "I am meditating" or "I am feeling this" or "I am free of thinking" or "I am being Reiki" or "I am in this state of emptiness and I like it," then this is just another thought; we are distracted by the present moment. This is where we lose being grateful. So therefore the precepts Do not anger and Do not worry are linked to the past and future. Being grateful has to do with the present.

We need to open up so we're not attached to any of these. So we are not carrying the past, not focusing on the future and not constantly analyzing this present moment. Then we can be really true to our way and our being. Through being true to our way and our being – compassion comes forward! Pure compassion. Pure compassion is something that already exists inside everybody. It's not something we have to acquire from the outside; it is our beautiful innate great bright light. It's like how water is wet. I cannot take the wetness out of water, right? So the quality of this innate great bright light is compassion. To have that pure compassion come forward, we need to let go of the past, the present and the future, or put simply – we have to let go of the three times.

This is really why we practice focusing, so that we do not get distracted by the three times. And we can see this within all five elements of the system of Reiki. We focus on the hands, or on a mantra, or on a symbol, we focus on the body, speech, mind aspects of the teachings, and we focus with the precepts. Each time we get distracted in our practice, in the form, we can ask, am I distracted by past, present and future? If so, we can refocus on the body, mind, speech aspect. The more we practice this, the more we can start to experience the no-form along with the form.

At that time your activity becomes Buddha's activity: time becomes supreme time, beyond any concept of past, present, or future; place becomes supreme place, beyond any dualistic concept; and person becomes supreme person, who is melted into the universe.
– Each Moment is the Universe: Zen and the Way of Being Time by Dainin Katagiri

Chapter 12:

Outcome of the Practice

We have looked at the foundations of the practice, looked at the physical aspects of how to practice, and how to create the right environment within ourselves for our practice. So now let's look at the outcome of our practice. Many people think that to practice the system of Reiki means that we become more intuitive or psychic, that we feel more energy, or we start to see auras... and some of that may be true for some people apart from their practice. But that is not the outcome at all. In fact for that, we do not have to practice that much. Just stick your finger in a power socket and you feel lots of energy. (Do not do this at home.) Or we just hit ourselves with an iron bar and we see lots of colors; also do not do this at home. But you get the idea. This is why we have to aim very clearly at what our target is, because what we aim at is what we are going to get out of the practice.

All of the five different elements in fact have the same aim, they all point towards the same thing: rediscovering our True Self. Do not get distracted by all the different practices. As we said before, that would be like getting distracted by the finger pointing at the moon, seeing the finger but not the moon. If we get distracted by the practices, then we can't see what the practices are pointing at. So then, how can we check to see how our personal practice is going? Do we look at how much energy we feel or how hot our hands are? Or how well someone feels after we have had a hands on/off healing session with them? No, we have to explore something very different.

Mikao Usui put pointers, guidelines, within his teachings to help us with questions like how our practice is going and what is the outcome of our practice. Some of these pointers are the precepts and the mantras. We can ask ourselves a few specific questions to see how our practice is going, but we have to be really honest with ourselves in our answers. Here are some of these questions:

How much ego clinging do we still have? Do we find that our ego clinging is softening through our practice?

Has our motivation changed since we started practicing? Do we practice just to feel energy or just for hands on/off healing, or is our motivation different now? And if so what is our motivation now?

How focused are we in our meditation practice? Is it sharp or dull? How is our meditation going? Are we distracted by the past, present, or future?

How are we conducting ourselves in daily life? Has this changed and if so how?

Has our practice become more natural?

Do we still have an agenda within our practice or can we let that go?

Do we have hopes and fears within our practice?

Have we become less self-centered?

Do we feel we have to sustain this spacious state of mind or does it feel like it carries on all by itself? Does sustaining it feel like "work", or can we return to our practice without judgement?

Let's look at, for example, hope and fear. Are we worried that we can't meditate, that we can't remember our True Self? Or are we attached to a specific outcome and can't let that go? In other words, how much hope and fear are we still holding on to? These are all important elements to contemplate if we want to create the right environment for our practice to blossom. And if we look carefully, we can see all of these are pointing towards the precepts.

Do not anger
Do not worry
Be grateful
Be true to your way and your being
Show compassion to yourself and others

And these contemplations are pointing towards what the mantras show us as well: a state of mind of interconnectedness and a blending of duality and non-duality. Thus real healing is about the direct experience of our True Self in all we do. That is the most compassionate thing we can do for ourselves, and for others. Because now we start to behave in a compassionate way towards others as well. In fact show compassion to yourself and others is all about the dissolving of the "I", then there is just compassion.

It is pretty hard to forget yourself and just help people. It takes time to learn this practice. But finally you touch the bottom of your life. This is the final stage. You forget yourself, and also you completely forget that you are sharing your life. You just stand back and support people without expecting anything, sometimes with silence, sometimes with words, sometimes with actions, sometimes with a laugh. This is peace – real peace.
– The Light That Shines Through Infinity by Dainin Katagiri

When we have a deeper experience of these elements – the precepts, the state of mind of interconnectedness, non-duality, emptiness – we can feel it within our mind, body, and energy; there's no doubt about that. But we also have to let go of attachments to these feelings and experiences. Let it all go. So it is great to check how our practice is going, because then we can see elements where we may want or need to adjust our practice and how we can adjust it. But we also have to let go of looking for an outcome, or as they say so simply and beautifully in

Japan: "Just Practice."

"Just practice" is like the bow and arrow: you aim and then you let go. But we have to notice what it is we are aiming at. Are you aiming at seeing colors or healing someone? Or are you aiming at the complete embodiment of the precepts in your daily life? These are very different aims and thus have different outcomes. We first must have a very clear idea about our aim. And then we have to let go, else the arrow will never hit the target. So examine your target, your aim, examine your practice and then let go and just practice.

If we are stuck always on an "I" this and an "I" that, putting ourselves in the center and expecting things to be the way we want them to be, we live always in a struggle between how we think things should be and how they are in fact different from that.
– Ten Ox Herding Pictures by Zen Master Shodo Harada

Part II:
Practicing

In the first part of the book we have looked at how to prepare ourselves to practice in the right way. If our practice is not perfect we also do not create the perfect fruit, and what is this fruit? It is a direct experience of our True Self in all we do. Therefore we first have to work with and understand the preparation so that when we now start with the practices, the soil is ripe and ready so that the plant can grow and our practice can bear fruit. And what is the seed that we put in the fertile soil? The seed of compassion, compassion for ourselves and others.

Here you have a match, and if you strike it a flame will appear. But if you don't know how to strike it, nothing will happen. The match is likened to honsho, original enlightenment. Striking it is likened to myoshu, excellent training.
– Discovering the True Self by Kōdō Sawaki

Before we delve further into how to practice, let's briefly recap the steps in the process. We use these points with each practice of the system of Reiki. Do all of this gently, not forcefully.

1 – Put your body in the right posture.
2 – Check your breathing, deep into the hara.
3 – Look at your mind and let go of clinging.
4 – Infuse your practice with emptiness – no-form.
5 – Mix in compassion; practice because you want to help others.
6 – Aim to remember your True Self; let go.
7 – Apply the method – form; just practice.
8 – During the practice let go of what comes up, with no clinging.
9 – Stay focused, not being distracted by past, present and future.
10 – Stop the method – form.
11 – Sit in that space of no-form, no distraction, no clinging.
12 – Move first your mind, speech and then your body, and progress with your day.

If you have started to think, "I am concentrating perfectly," then your concentration has already stopped, your individual self exists again, and you don't see your real self.
– The Light That Shines Through Infinity by Dainin Katagiri

Chapter 13:

Shoden Reiki I

The following chapters explain the essential practices of the three levels of the system of Reiki from a Japanese perspective. There is no need to add more; the system of Reiki is perfect just the way Mikao Usui created it, as a way to rediscovering our True Self. The more we add, the more we get confused about what to practice and the more we remove ourselves from the path towards non-duality. So whatever we practice, let's make sure the aim is non-duality. We are already soaked in duality and we all know how this has been working out so far for the world: confusion, hate, worry, fear, division, you name it. Thus whatever we practice, let's practice it with the mindset of non-duality. Because it is only through this that we start to have real compassion for each being, equally.

Shoden means beginning teachings and thus it is the beginning of our journey of self-discovery, rediscovering our non-dual nature, the great bright light, our True Self. As it is the beginning we need to make sure we build a solid foundation and that is really what the practices are about at this level. Hence it is better to work with these practices for a prolonged amount of time so that the foundation becomes really solid. Again, if the foundation is not solid the house might collapse later on. If the ground is not made fertile, the plant will not bear fruit and maybe it will wither.

The Precepts

Everyone knows how much anger hurts people, so we should stay calm and not be angry. But when we face anger, we are completely at a loss over what to do. Finally we fight. That is why again and

again – forever – we have to listen for the truth and think deeply how we keep the precepts in everyday life. Constantly explore the meaning of the precepts through your practice.
– The Light That Shines Through Infinity by Dainin Katagiri

The first element we learn within Shoden Reiki I is the precepts, as they are the foundation of the whole system. Therefore, a deep and solid understanding of the precepts is essential for all the other practices to rest upon. The precepts are a wonderful tool to lay bare our True Self; they are in fact a description of our True Self. In an earlier chapter, we looked closely at the meaning of the precepts. But how can we use the precepts within our practice, with the aim of non-duality? The first practice element is contemplation; we contemplate the precepts.

Do not anger
Do not worry
Be grateful
Practice diligently – Be true to your way and your being
Show compassion to yourself and others

How do we contemplate? We ask ourselves questions like, who is this "I" who gets angry and worried? Can I find this "I"? Does it have a shape, and so on. When we do this kind of practice, this self-inquiry, often we come to a conclusion that we cannot find the "I"; the "I" is just a human construct and is not our True Self. But we have to be utterly sure about it. Through this we see that the "I" is linked to our name, our body and our mind. But our body is not the "I" and neither is the mind. Our name is just some letters and therefore also is not the "I". Through this kind of investigation we can start to soften the grip on the "I". We also can soften this grip by examining our thoughts.

When we examine our thoughts, we have to look at where they came from, where they reside, and where are they going.

Can we find the source of our thoughts, whether they are happy or angry thoughts? Through thorough investigation, we see that these thoughts have no base, no roots so to speak; they will come and they will go. We start to get glimpses of emptiness, our True Self, the wide open spaciousness of our mind. Through doing this kind of practice, we begin to find a clarity in which we can see a thought arising but now we do not cling to the thought. And therefore the thought dissolves all by itself. And maybe the thought that arises next is an answer to a question we have or a solution to an issue we need to address. Because by not clinging to a thought, we have more open space for clarity in our mind.

We realize that our True Self is like the bright blue wide open sky and that the clouds are our thoughts, and that we do not have to follow the thoughts. With practice, we can learn how to rest our mind just on the wide open sky, our True Self. Then clouds come and go all by themselves and we are not attached to them. Don't pursue the thought; when we pursue the thought we are stretching the thought out and therefore also our pain and discomfort. This is in reality also true with a happy thought, because now we cling to happiness and if this suddenly changes we start to get angry and worried again. We have to rediscover that we are not our thoughts. When I lived in the Himalayas I heard a story of old masters who were kind of singing to themselves: "Mind do not wander, mind do not wander," as a reminder to themselves to stay mindful.

When performing the meditation practice one should develop the feeling of opening oneself completely to the whole universe with absolute simplicity and nakedness of mind, ridding oneself of all protecting barriers. Don't mentally split into two when meditating, one part of the mind watching the other like a cat watching a mouse. One should realize that one does not meditate to go deeply within oneself and withdraw from the world: complete

openness of mind is the essential point.
– Dilgo Khyentse Rinpoche

But this kind of practice is not for everybody; we have to find what suits our disposition. This is why Mikao Usui had no standard curriculum and his teachings would depend on the spiritual disposition of each student.

Here is another practice which we can do with the precepts; we can chant them. We already have seen this instruction within the full text of the precepts, remember:

Morning and evening perform gassho
Keep in your mind
Chant with your mouth

The best way is to chant the precepts in Japanese, and while we chant there is no need to contemplate them; just chant. This is not a contemplation practice; this is just chanting.

Kyo dake wa
Ikaru-na
Shinpai suna
Kansha shite
Gyo o hage me
Hito ni shin-setsu ni

We have to chant the precepts from our hara and this is why our body posture and breathing is so important. When we start to chant this in the right way we will ignite the inner fire within our body. But this doesn't happen instantaneously; it takes time. This is why we aim and let go. Let go of any hopes and fears, expectations that it might happen and fears that it might not happen at all. When we let go of hope and fear, we are in fact laying bare more spaciousness and we all know that fire needs space to burn. Do not try to memorize them because if we try to chant from memory and then we forget, we may get angry with ourselves and this is of course counterproductive. Just print them out and read them while you chant. Reading while we chant creates an extra focus point. If we chant them by rote and our mind is getting distracted by the past, present, and future during the chanting then we are not getting the desired results. Because we can only really discover our True Self when we do not cling to all those thoughts. This is why we have to be mindful during the practices, mindful of not being distracted.

We do not need to train in distraction, as we are that during our daily life already; we need to train in not being distracted. Hence if we let our mind just wander during any of the practice, we train our self in even more distraction and how can we then be non-distracted in our daily life? Impossible. Thus be mindful during the practice, not being distracted by past, present, and future, and if the mind wanders, gently bringing it back to focus. Because it is only through this that we start to lay bare our True Self, our essence.

Use your mouth when you chant. Do not just mumble the word; chant it deeply from within and let it resonate through your whole physical body. Through this resonance we can slowly dislodge all the stuck trauma and energy in our body and energy system so that we create the right environment for that fire, mist, and rain to take place: inner transformation. Our body is like the alchemical vessel in which we create transformation, transformation from being confused and distracted all the time to a compassionate human being who is focused and centered, full of love and kindness. This kind of compassion is a compassion which does not change. Normally, if we are kind to this person but not that person, to this group but not that group, our kindness is changeable. But real compassion does not change; it is unchangeable because it comes from emptiness.

When you chant, be as empty as possible, imagine a singing

bowl, it only resonates so well due to being empty. If you put some socks into the singing bowl the sound will be not so pure. Thus to be able to have that really direct experience, be empty during the chanting. In fact be empty during any of the practices as taught within the system of Reiki; only then do we create the right ripple effect.

If you want to hear the precepts chanted in Japanese, you can Google "Frans Stiene chanting precepts".

Meditation Practices

The second element we learn in Shoden Reiki I is the breath meditation practices, which are the foundation of hands on/off healing on ourselves and others. The first of these meditation practices is jōshin kokyū hō. (Of course all the other practices are also meditation practices!)

Meditation not only makes your spiritual energy stronger but also cures illnesses and helps to get rid of fatigue.

– Reiki Ryôhô no Shiori which is handed out by the Usui Reiki Ryôhô Gakkai

Jōshin kokyū hō:

淨   jō means clear, pure, without taint or defilement, lucid

心   shin means heart, mind, essence, the mind as the principle of the universe, the enlightened mind

呼吸 kokyū means to exhale and inhale, breathing

法   hō means method, dharma, principle

We therefore can translate jōshin kokyū hō in this way: The method to rediscovering our pure mind through breathing.

So here Mikao Usui again points out our pure mind, like within the precepts, and reminds us that we have to rediscover it. What is that pure mind? Emptiness, our great bright light. Both the meditation practices and the precepts point to the mind, because this is the essence of Mikao Usui's teachings. This pure mind is called anshin ritsumei in Japan, which means peace of mind. Why peace of mind? Because we are not distracted by the past, present, and future; we are not clinging to our thoughts. Through this practice we learn to rest our mind in our pure mind which is emptiness, freedom.

Practicing jōshin kokyū hō:

1. Sit and gassho.
2. Place your hands in your lap, palms facing upwards.
3. With each in-breath, feel/visualize a bright energy coming in through the nose and bring it down to the hara, just below your navel. When you do this, link the visual with the breath and the mind.
4. Feel/visualize the bright energy, the breath and the mind expanding through your body.
5. On the out-breath, expand the bright energy, the breath and the mind out of the body, through your skin, out into infinity.
6. Repeat steps 3 to 5 until finished.

The secret of sustaining life and attaining longevity is found in disciplining the body. The secret of disciplining the body is to focus the mind in the tanden [hara] located in the ocean of ki. When the mind focuses in the tanden, ki gathers there. When ki gathers in the tanden, the true elixir is produced. When the elixir is produced, the physical frame is strong and firm and the life-force is full and replete. When the life-force is full and replete, longevity is assured. This corresponds to the secret method that the ancient sages perfected for "refining the elixir nine times over" and "returning it to the source." You must know that the elixir is not

something located apart from the self. The essential concern above all else is to make the fire or heat in your mind (heart) descend into the lower body so that it fills the tanden in the ocean of ki.
– Hakuin's Precious Mirror Cave by Norman Waddell

It looks simple but we have to keep in mind some very important elements. Remember to include in this practice all the other elements we have discussed before: compassion, form and no-form, mind-body-speech... if it helps, as you are beginning your practice, you might look back at the Contents or make a list. When we link the mind with the breath and use the body as the base, we create a solid focus. In the Asian meditation tradition this is called samatha, which means calming the mind. With the in-breath into the hara, we train ourselves in being mindful, not distracted by the past, present, and future, as we solely focus on the breath. When we breathe out into infinity and we feel this union with the universe, that is vipassana, which means insight, or clear seeing.

What are we clearly seeing? We are seeing (in time, with practice) our pure mind, non-duality, emptiness, our great bright light. This specific meditation is based on ancient Tendai Buddhist meditations and can still be found in their traditions. This is not surprising. As every school of Reiki teaches its beginning students, Mikao Usui meditated on Mount Kurama for 21 days. And at that time, the main temple on Mount Kurama, Kurama-dera, belonged to the Tendai Buddhist sect. But as all these ancient teachings point out, we need first to calm the mind until we can have a clear insight into our True Self. Do not get caught up during practice by what you feel, see, sense, or do not feel, see, sense... that is a distraction and therefore we are not calming the mind at all. It stays busy; that is not the perfect way to practice and thus it will not create a fertile ground to bear the right fruit of our practice.

In short, all this should emphasize the concentration of power in the whole body by simultaneously placing strength in the tanden [hara] and by infusing the whole body with energy moving away from the tanden. Thus, by means of the equilibrium of the centrifugal and the centripetal force, the whole body is brought to a state of zero and spiritual power will pervade the whole body intensely.
– Introduction to Zen Training: A Physical Approach to Meditation and Mind-Body Training by Omori Sogen

Also, can you see sanmitsu – mind, body, speech – within this practice? We place the body in the right posture, we use the breath, we use a visual for the mind aspect; hence this practice is a perfect sanmitsu practice.

Let's briefly touch upon samatha and vipassana. In reality it doesn't matter what we name these qualities, but it is important to understand them and why they are important. If we can focus one-pointedly, thus not being distracted, we have samatha. Not easy, right? This is why Mikao Usui put all the focus practices within his system, the form practices, so that we can learn how to be mindful, how to stay focused. Vipassana is seeing the truth, universal truth, that there is no "I", and thus no "you" and "me". Or in other words, seeing our True Self. In many of these teachings you mix samatha focus practice with vipasyana insight practice, just like in jōshin kokyū hō.

When samatha is developed, one eliminates distracting thoughts that keep one from being able to examine or analyze things. Removing the distraction of thoughts leads to perceiving things very clearly and distinctly, which is vipašyaná.
– The Practice of Tranquillity and Insight by Khenchen Thrangu

In samatha practices you have samatha with an external support; we focus on something external like a statue or candle. And you have samatha with internal support, the breath for example, just like in jōshin kokyū hō. But as the breath is more subtle than an external support it might be a bit harder for people to focus on, and therefore there are also slightly different versions of jōshin kokyū hō. These versions are a bit more physical, so that we can rest the mind on the body which is not as subtle as the breath. A good Reiki teacher will be able to help you with this.

Seishin toitsu:

The next meditation practice we learn is seishin toitsu. And again we see that this is the perfect sanmitsu practice, as we use the body, mind, and breath again. This practice is really a samatha practice, as it teaches us pure focus. It teaches us not being distracted.

精	sei = polish – refine – pure – undiluted – clear – effort – essence – essential
神	shin = spiritual power – incredible – kami – deity
精神	seishin = mind, essence, consciousness, intention
統	toi = to gather into one – the whole – unification
一	tsu = one
統一	toitsu = unity – unification, harmony

Seishin toitsu also points out the pure nature of our mind, as jōshin kokyū hō does, and that we have to gather our mind into one. Normally our mind is all over the place: past, present, and future. To gather our mind into one means to realize emptiness, non-duality, and we do this through concentration. Seishin toitsu therefore also stands for concentration, and we cannot concentrate if we are unfocused, if we are distracted by our mind chatter.

In Japanese, concentration is called Seishin Toitsu. Seishin is a pure mind, or the spirit. Toitsu is gathering together, or focusing on the here and now. Basically it means that the mind is focused toward achieving the task at hand. This unity of mind and body, spirit and action, is the same as giving total effort. It is only when a person is centered and focused that one can act decisively, as is required in Judo.

– Concentration in Judo Training by Neil Ohlenkamp

Practicing seishin toitsu:

1. With your hands in the gassho position, focus on your hara. On the in-breath, begin to bring the energy/breath and mind into your fingertips – hands. Feel the energy/breath and mind move through your arms, down through your body and into the hara.

2. On the out-breath, visualize energy/breath and mind moving from the hara back up through the body and then to the arms and out through the hands – fingertips.

Again this looks very simple but there are many hidden layers to this practice. Thus remember the preparation again, and each time you get distracted bring your mind back to the practice. Energy follows the mind so it is important to do this practice correctly, else the energy will not go to your hara because your mind is somewhere else. Concentrate. The mind is inside the body, as we also want to soften and purify the meridians in our hands, arms, and the central channel of our body. We do this so that the inner fire which we have awakened within the hara can gradually start to move through our whole energy system. This in turn will burn all our dualistic ideas and thus will help us to lay bare our True Self.

To be able to do these meditation practices well, we need to check during the practice that we are not falling asleep. If we do, if we start to feel drowsy, then we might think our practice is going well because we are not following our thoughts. But it only feels that way; an undercurrent of thoughts still is taking place, but because there is no clarity we are not aware of them. If this happens, lift the head a bit upwards, open the eyes slightly and even look upwards so that the drowsiness disappears. There also are times, maybe often, when we are too distracted in our practice and we feel like we cannot focus the mind. Then look downwards, tilt the head a bit downwards as well; in doing this we can create more stability. Our meditation needs to be clear: no clarity no focus, no fruition.

Kenyokū hō:

乾　ken = dry, clean
浴　yoku = bathe
法　ho = dharma, ultimate truth, method

Temizu-no-gi (washing of hands and mouth).The first ritual is performed at the temizuya, the ablution pavilion at the entrance to the precincts. A small ladle (haidatsu) with a long handle is used. Water is scooped from a trough of running water and, with the ladle held in the right hand, a little is poured over the left. The ladle is then transferred to the left hand and the right hand is similarly washed. Thereafter, returning the ladle to the right hand, more water is poured on the left hand, some of which is taken into the mouth. This is emptied in front of the trough, the ladle is rinsed, and the ritual is completed. The worshipper may now proceed to the shrine precincts proper.
– Essentials of Shinto: An Analytical Guide to Principal Teachings by Stuart D.B. Picken

This method of dry bathing is also a meditation practice, which means we have to do it mindfully. If we are distracted, without focus, we will not get the deeper benefit from this practice. Dry bathing means that we do not use water, but just imagine if we are using water. If we do not focus the shower head on our body, we might take a shower but the water will never reach our body, hence we lose the benefit of having a shower. Thus, do this practice with supreme focus, not being distracted by past, present, and future. This also means that we have to stroke the body physically, breathing into the hara, else we also lose the desired effect. If we do not stroke ourselves physically, it will be the same as not focusing the shower head; the water never reaches our body.

Practicing kenyokū hō:

1. Gassho – to center the mind and set intent while standing or sitting.
2a. Place your right hand on the left shoulder. Breathe into the hara, and on the out-breath, sweep diagonally down from the left shoulder to the right hip.
2b. On the in-breath into the hara, place your left hand on the right shoulder and, on the out-breath, sweep down diagonally from right shoulder to left hip.
2c. Breathe into the hara, returning your right hand to the left shoulder and, on the out-breath, sweep diagonally down from left shoulder to right hip.
3a. On the next in-breath into the hara, place your right hand on the left shoulder; on the out-breath, sweep downward along the arm to the fingertips, palm facing upwards.
3b. On the next in-breath into the hara, place your left hand on the right shoulder; on the out-breath, sweep downward along the arm to the fingertips, palm facing upwards.
3c. On the next in-breath into the hara, place your right hand on the left shoulder; on the out-breath, sweep downward along the arm to the fingertips, palm facing upwards.

There are slightly different versions of this practice, in which you sweep from elbow to fingertips. But as one of the aims is to really clear the meridians in your arms and torso, it is better to stroke the whole arm.

Dry bathing has its roots in ancient Shinto, often used with water, and falls under the heading of misogi, which stands for purification. What are we purifying? We are purifying our confused mind. This practice is very much about the union of body-mind and that is why we focus on the physical body. This practice is not about sweeping away energy which you have picked up from somewhere; that is dualistic thinking. This practice is really about laying bare our pure mind of non-duality. Remember the aim: if we keep practicing with the idea of duality in our mind, we never lay bare our non-dual nature; it will be impossible.

Misogi is a washing away of all defilements, a removal of all obstacles, a separation from disorder, an abstention from negative thought, a radiant state of unadorned purity, the accomplishment of all things, a condition of lofty virtue, and a spotless environment. In misogi one returns to the very beginning, where there is no differentiation between oneself and the universe.
– Founder of Aikido, Morihei Ueshiba

We can use this practice as a standalone method or we can use it before or after we do a hands on/off healing session. We can use it before or after we perform reiju, before and after we do seishin toitsu, and so on. It all depends on how our mind is: clear and centered, or distracted. Again, this practice is not about duality, sweeping away negative energy picked up outside of ourselves. This practice is about being stable in our body, centered and yet open, remembering our non-dual nature. And from that state of openness we perform, for example, hands on/off healing. Then why do we do it after the hands on/off healing session? Because maybe during the hands on/off healing we have become ungrounded due to experiencing a lot of energy and openness. Thus we have to bring our mind into our body again, stabilizing and anchoring ourselves.

Hands on/off Healing on Ourselves

Ritual depends on your attitude and behaviour.
— The Light That Shines Through Infinity by Dainin Katagiri

Finally we have hands on/off healing on ourselves and others within Shoden Reiki I. But again this really comes from a stable mind, body, and energy. And therefore the previous meditation practices are the foundation for hands on/off healing. Without this stability we can become, to name just a few, unfocused, worried, angry, or fearful. In many modern Reiki schools they say "we practice Reiki" as a means of saying that they practice hands on/off healing. But as it is just one element of the system of Reiki, in Japan hands on/off healing is not called Reiki; it is called teate or tenohira – palm healing.

We have a word "teate" in Japanese (literally means put hand on injury). When we feel ill, we put our hands on the part of the body that hurts naturally. At that time, we never push too hard on the painful place. You just send your mind (Ki) to the place where you experience pain. To put it plainly, this is Kiatsu therapy.
— Ki Breathing by Koichi Tohei

The practice of hands on/off healing is also a meditation practice, although that fact is not taught in many modern Reiki courses. That actually is a shame as it means the people offering these courses misunderstand this particular element of Mikao Usui's teachings. Remember, energy follows the mind; thus if our mind is distracted during hands on/off healing, our energy also is distracted. This is why in Mikao Usui's time, this practice always was considered a meditative practice. We can very easily check this; if we are angry all day, do we feel tired or not? If we are worried all day, do we feel tired or not? Of course we do. Why? Because our anger and worry have eaten up our energy.

Thus the energy has followed our distracted, worried and angry mind, to the future and the past.

The point is to introduce and emphasize the very strong Japanese feeling that one's whole being (physical form and mental attitude) is so inseparably connected that one can train the mind-aspect by focusing upon the body-aspect. Indeed, this is the easiest way to train the mind-aspect since it is invisible and without shape, color, and form. The body-aspect, on the other hand, may easily be disciplined under the supervision of a master. Accordingly, even in religious practice, the body serves as a vehicle for, not a detriment to, the direct experience of the highest religious truth.

– The Bodymind Experience in Japanese Buddhism: A Phenomenological Study of Kukai and Dogen by David Edward Shaner

In his instructions, the precepts, Mikao Usui pointed out mind, body, energy. As we can see in the above quote, the body is a perfect tool for training the mind. The mind is very subtle and the breath/energy also is more subtle than our body, thus harder to grasp. We also can see this within Yoga or Tai Chi, for example: you use your body to regulate your mind and energy. But to be able to do this we need to stay focused, mindful, during hands on/off healing. If we are not mindful, if we are unfocused, distracted by the past, present, and future, then hands on/off healing will not be a practice to train the mind because we are not including the mind in the practice! We are only using the body, the hands. Please do remember this. This is very important, especially if we want to see Mikao Usui's teachings as a path to anshin ritsumei, a calm and peaceful mind.

Some groups claim that 臼井霊気療法 Usui Reiki Ryôhô was intended to cure disease, as the Japanese word 療法 "Ryôhô" literally means the curing therapy. If so, Usui Reiki Ryôhô would

have been just another one of the treatment therapies that existed before Usui Sensei. Usui Sensei said, "I have never studied any methods for disease treatment." He also stated, "Usui Reiki Ryôhô makes us fit and well, moderates our thought and enhances one's joy of life," and "Usui Reiki Ryôhô heals Kokoro [mind and spirit] first, and then makes the body strong and healthy." These statements of his clearly mean that he did not give first priority to curing disease. Usui Sensei wrote two descriptive statements that introduce 五戒 Go-kai The Five Precepts: 招福の秘法 "Shofuku no Hiho" "The secret method to invite happiness" and the second one, 萬病の霊薬 "Manbyo no Reiyaku" "The miraculous remedy/elixir for all diseases" that follows it. In this way he indicates that the ultimate goal of Usui Reiki Ryôhô is to become happy and that we enter this happy state by becoming healthy through hand healing.
– Hiroshi Doi

In this book I am not going to offer you a specific set of hand positions; the "standard" positions often taught are widely available. Hands on/off healing in essence needs to be natural and flowing; each person is different and therefore is in need of different hand positions. A good acupuncturist would not stick the needles in every person in the same spots, would they? Instead I will teach you the proper way of hands on/off healing as Mikao Usui pointed out in his teachings.

Let's first discuss hands on/off healing on ourselves, as this is the base for helping others. If we do not know how to correctly perform hands on/off healing on ourselves, then how can we perform it correctly on others? Thus we first have to experiment on and with ourselves to see what is the truth. This might not be clear in one session, but if we do a 20 minute session each day for a few months one way, with a focused mind, and then another way, with a distracted mind, it will become very obvious what that truth is.

What was Mikao Usui pointing out again as the main aim?

A peaceful mind, emptiness, our great bright light; thus that is already the aim of hands on/off healing. This is how we start with this practice. Our aim is not healing a pain in our knee; that is really a side effect of remembering our True Self, a peaceful mind. Because when my mind is peaceful, energy, ki, will flow freely through my whole body. If my mind is stuck in the past, present, and future then my energy is also stuck.

If ki is extended throughout the entire body and there is no stagnation, there is no defect/illness. If ki is dispersed and becomes diminished, there is defect/illness. Indeed, if ki is diminished, energy becomes weak, [ki] will not be able to circulate, [ki] will become stagnant here and there, and a defect/illness will form.
– Isetsu 醫 説 *(Discourse on Medicine) by Takuan Soho (1573-1645)*

Zen master Takuan Soho explains it perfectly; when our ki is extended through our entire body there is no illness, but when our ki becomes dispersed/scattered, there will be illness. When is our ki dispersed? When we get distracted by the past, present, future, when we are not resting our mind in emptiness. Thus if we practice hands on/off healing with a distracted mind, then we only create more dispersed energy, and our energy is not freely extended through our entire body! This is why it is of utmost importance to focus during hands on/off healing.

Thus when we start hands on/off healing on ourselves, it might be better first to sit in a chair, straight, so that we can stay focused. Often people do this lying down but then we may fall asleep. And when we fall asleep we are also distracted; our dreams take us here and there and everywhere. Thus start sitting. Again, remember the preparation elements: checking our mind, body, and breath, emptiness, compassion... review them when you need to. Never forget these important ingredients of the practice; they are essential. No water and sunshine on a plant: no growth, no fruit. Of course if we see hands on/off healing as just a relaxation method, there's no need to do this preparation. But if we want to relax, we might just as well take a nap; it's easy, costs less, and we do not have to take a course to learn how to do it. Relaxation is a wonderful by-product of the practice, but it is not what Mikao Usui's teachings are about. It is about rediscovering our True Self, our peaceful mind.

Now start to place the hands on/off the body, focus your mind on the hands, and each time the mind drifts towards the past, present, future, bring the mind back to the hands. Do this for 10, 20, 45 minutes or even two minutes. But of course the more we train our mind to be focused, the more freely our energy flows through our body, and the deeper the healing will be.

Some Reiki schools teach methods of only hands off the body and some say on the body; it's better to do both. But unless there is a good reason not to – for example, an area is too painful to touch, or trauma associated with touch is too deep – on the body is the best. Why? Because we make friends with our body, we feel the hands on our physical body, so we start to be more in the body too. And when we touch the physical body, we also soften the energy lines and centers in our body, so it's more direct, so to speak. Plus when we feel our hands touching ourselves something else starts to take place; the more we feel this physical touch the more we realize that we are the giver and the receiver at the same time! Through this experience, we start to soften the grip on the "I". Why?

Because normally we either are the giver or we are the receiver. But with physical hands on healing on our body, we are very clearly the giver and the receiver at the same time. This softens the dual concept and therefore helps us to enter that state of non-duality. But we have to stay focused to be able to do this. Now hands on healing becomes a samatha meditation practice. As pointed out before, we do not have to train our mind into distraction – that is easy, and we do it all the time. But we do have to train the mind into non-distraction, supreme focus. This means that if we practice daily a focused hands on healing session, samatha, we are meditating daily. And therefore it becomes easier to lay bare clear insight, vipasyana, our True Self.

If you see something wonderful through your practice, you may attach to what you have seen because it was a valuable experience for you. But when you are caught by the idea of what you experienced, it becomes a problem for you.

– The Light That Shines Through Infinity by Dainin Katagiri

This also means not to get distracted by what we feel, experience, sense or see. As soon as we say to ourselves, "this is hot", "this is cold", "this means this and that means that", "I see purple; what does that mean?", then we are distracted. We are distracted by the present moment. And when we are distracted by the present moment, we have moved away from our True Self, from that peaceful mind. Thus when we occupy ourselves with these kinds of ideas, these interpretations, we are training ourselves for distraction instead of focus. And that in itself is counterproductive to what the practice is really about, taming the wild monkey mind so that our energy will be free and flowing.

Hands on/off Healing on Others

The ordinary idea of "observing" is to see something in the distance. This is dualistic. Real observing is to merge, to become one with, the dynamic process of observation itself. How can we understand this? According to grammatical structure, a sentence is made up of subject, object, and verb. But when you, as the subject, exactly participate in your object, then your object is not something separate from you. You are exactly the same and one –

101

so there is no object. If there is no object, very naturally there can be no subject. What's left? The verb! Activity itself!
– The Light That Shines Through Infinity by Dainin Katagiri

To do hands on/off healing on others, we have to let go of the dualistic idea; we have to just become touch, the activity of touch itself. This is when we have let go of object "I", subject "you", and thus all that is left is the verb, the activity itself. But we can only rediscover that when first we work on ourselves. After we have worked on ourselves, not just with hands on/off healing, but also with chanting the precepts, contemplating the "I", and practicing the meditation methods, we can start to do hands on/off healing on others. The base for helping others is to have a calm peaceful centered state of mind. Else we mix, for example, worry and fear into our hands on/off healing on others.

Moving with that mysterious functioning where there is no separation between the person who is helping and the person who is being helped.
– Ten Ox Herding Pictures by Zen Master Shodo Harada

When we perform hands on/off healing on others as an act of meditation, then the practice itself becomes a practice for realizing our True Self, realizing that there is no separation between the person who is helping and the person who is being helped – non-duality. But again, this can only take place when we take the "I" out of the practice. Hence when we practice hands on/off healing on others and we are constantly analyzing: "I feel this", "I see something", "I", "I", "I", then that direct experience of non-duality of non-separation cannot and will not take place. This is why we also start hands on/off healing on others with mind, body, breath, focus, with emptiness and compassion... so that now hands on/off healing on others becomes a fertile ground for our great bright light to manifest, and not an exercise in distraction by past, present, and future. When we start to perform hands on/off healing like this, our whole act will be an act of pure compassion rising out of emptiness, no strings attached to the session, pure openness, just touch.

Seeing that our fears do nothing but restrict our energy can give us tremendous power and strength, enabling us to discover the true dynamism of our consciousness. Nothing in the physical world can protect us from objects of fear; transcending fear itself through meditation is our true protection.
– Openness Mind: Self-Knowledge and Inner Peace Through Meditation by Tarthang Tulku

Many people who start to perform hands on/off healing on others have not done enough preparation to be in the hara and to stabilize themselves. In return, this makes them want to protect themselves, as they feel overwhelmed by emotions, feelings they might have picked up. But in essence, and I am sorry to say this, that means that they are not ready yet to work on others. To be able to work on others, we need to be stable. Because if we feel the need to protect ourselves from others, we are building a barrier between each other, and this in itself is not conductive to healing. Plus when we go home we might feel overwhelmed, fearful, or any number of things. And this is not beneficial for ourselves. Hence it is better to first practice on our own so that we become stable like a mountain; a mountain is solid at the bottom, stable, and wide open at the top. Except for the letter in its name, a mountain has no "I". And the "I" is what creates the barrier, creates the problem.

Anytime you start a sentence with "I am" you are creating what you are and what you want to be.
– Dr. Wayne Dyer

I am an empath and therefore I pick things up.
I am an empath and need to protect myself.
I am super sensitive so please do not say these things.
I am a sensitive person so I feel a lot of pain from others.
I am a psychic and need to close my aura for protection.
I am a psychic and I pick up other people's pain.

This is why in Shoden Reiki I, we straight away have to explore the precepts, our great bright light, emptiness, compassion, our mind, body, and energy. Because it is through this exploration that we soften the habit of identifying ourselves with the "I".

But that of course is not easy; we love to focus on the "I", as that is how we "I"dentify ourselves. That is how we portray ourselves to others and, maybe even more so, to ourselves. This is who "I am", "I" have always been like this, "I" have always been sensitive or an empath or a psychic. But when we investigate this properly we realize that we are not the "I". The "I" we think we are is just a cloud in the stainless sky. Our True I, the True Self is the sky and is free of labels. Thus we have to rediscover our True I, which is stable, open and expanded, full of compassion and kindness without the need for protection. Like Wayne Dyer points out, as soon as we start a sentence with "I am" we are already creating what we are and what we want to be. We are in fact saying that we are picking things up, that we feel things and therefore we need to protect ourselves, that we are overwhelmed by all the senses and by what we pick up. Letting go of the "I", ego, is not that easy. But the first step we can take on the journey of our healing is to change the way we say things. Words matter. So instead of saying things like the statements above, we could change it to:

I am strong and centered.
I am balanced and whole.
I am clear and focused.

Of course these are just stepping stones to becoming whole, balanced, and clear. It is a small way of change, as we are still clinging to an "I". But we have to start somewhere.

The most direct way is to cut straight to the root of the problem and lay bare our essence: emptiness. But that is also not so easy; that is why we apply the methods of practice so this becomes a direct experience and embodiment, the embodiment of the letting go of the "I", ego. In fact when we lay bare emptiness, we start to realize that this "I" never existed in the first place. We can move toward this through practicing the meditation methods taught within the system of Reiki. But we need to keep on as we are holding on so tightly to the "I", ego, that it might take some years of practice to soften that grip. Words matter. Becoming whole, balanced and clear matters even more.

Watch your thoughts, they become your words; watch your words, they become your actions; watch your actions, they become your habits; watch your habits, they become your character; watch your character, it becomes your destiny.

– Lao Tzu

This is why it is also essential not to judge, label, and distinguish during a hands on/off healing session; let it all go. Some Reiki traditions focus on a practice called byosen reikan ho, a practice of sensing; however, this practice has been completely misunderstood. Often when we first learn hands on/off healing, we learn a strict protocol of hand positions. Thus the logical next step would be to become more flexible in this, more in-tune so to speak. Hence the practice of byosen reikan ho, becoming more flexible with our hand positions, tailor-making it for our clients as in reality each client is unique and each moment is unique. But then people started to label, distinguish, and analyze what they felt and here they got caught with the ego, the "I". "I" feel this and therefore it means that. But they misunderstood one very important element.

The Japanese word to describe the overall feeling of what you experience during byosen reikan ho is called hibiki. And hibiki means echo. What is an echo? Empty; it is pure emptiness. Getting caught up with an echo is like standing on a rock cliff and speaking back to the echo of your own voice as if it is another person talking to you. This is really called confusion and it creates confusion. Now we also understand why it is so important to understand the system of Reiki from its traditional Japanese perspective and why Mikao Usui used specific words and not others. They are all teachings, pointing us in the direction of emptiness. But again, we get confused by the finger pointing instead of looking at what it is pointing at, where it is pointing to.

Touch

Let's explore touch a bit more, as it is important to understand this within the scope of hands on/off healing on ourselves and others. But how do we touch? We have explored some of it already but other aspects are important as well. We already have seen that when we touch it is important that we have the right state of mind. Because if our mind is not in the right space, touch can become very different, even hurtful.

In the context of healing, we need to touch ourselves with the intent that we receive whatever we need, from a place of emptiness. There is no need to have a very specific, boxed-in intent, like "this or that needs to be healed"; in truth we do not really know what we need. We might think we do, but if we look honestly at ourselves we do not really know. So by setting a very open intent, from that state of emptiness, non-clinging, our mind and energy also become more open and thus allow a more free flowing energy. For example, say we have a pain in our knee. If we just touch our knee with the intent that our knee gets healed, we are setting a limited intent. And thus our touch is limiting, because maybe the pain in our knee comes from our sciatic nerve. And that issue might come from a tightness in our kidneys due to pent-up anger. If we set a more open intent when we touch our knee, the healing can take place on a much deeper level and our touch becomes something very different. In our daily life, we often are told by our parents or by society not to touch ourselves; thus we have created an obstacle through which our mind and energy don't flow. Touching our own body can be very healing and freeing. But again, we need to touch it with the right state of mind. What is this state of mind? This is the state of mind of no anger and worry or fear, a state of mind in which we are grateful for how our body looks and feels no matter what. And we have to couple our touch with our innate love and compassion. Therefore, if our touch is without anger, worry and fear, and is infused with gratefulness and compassion, then we have the right touch. By being mindful when we touch ourselves, which means our mind is not being distracted by past, present and future issues, we are therefore completely focused and open at the same time when we touch. This kind of touch, due to it being completely free, brings a deep kind of healing, peace and even inner joy and bliss. This kind of touch also helps us to accept our body.

First accept your human body, and then use it to manifest something more than what you understand – something deep.
– The Light That Shines Through Infinity by Dainin Katagiri

Recalling the precept be grateful, the first thing we have to be grateful of is our human body, for that is the vehicle in which we can realize our True Self. No human body, no direct experience of our True Self. Thus through touching ourselves we start to become grateful for our own body.

And thus, through knowing and learning how to touch ourselves with the right state of mind, we learn how to touch others when we perform a hands on/off healing session, or just in our daily life.

When we touch someone during a hands on/off session, we need to touch without anger, worry and fear and in a state of mind of gratitude and compassion. Often people touch with the intent of a specific outcome: that the person might be healed, feels something, has no more pain, or is happy. But in reality, this mindset comes from worry and fear; we may worry and fear that the client is not healed, does not feel anything, or still has pain and is not happy. If our mind is completely free of any specific intent, it therefore is completely open, emptiness. In this place of openness, we can touch the person in a spacious state of mind. This means that the space is so open that the energy can flow freely through both practitioner and client without any obstacles. This in turn creates a deep state of mind for healing to take place, and even for inner joy and bliss to occur.

When we first start to experience this kind of deeper touch, it might start to feel very intimate. So to be able to do this kind of touching we need to stay centered and grounded. This kind of intimacy has nothing to do with sex; rather it is a remembering that the person who is touching is also being touched at the same time! Thus during this kind of touching, a mutual state of healing will take place. This kind of touching is also very important if we want to keep our relationship healthy with our partner. Often we may touch our partner, when we make love for example, in a distracted state of mind. Our mind is not focused and open. It is thinking about the past, present and future. But when our mind lets go of the past, present, and future, our touch becomes something very different. Now it is devoid of anger, worry, and fear; it is infused with gratitude and compassion. This kind of lovemaking can trigger deep forms of inner joy and bliss which will heal many wounds that are often created in relationships. When we touch each other like this during our lovemaking, then lovemaking becomes magical and healing. Something very deep and intimate takes place between two people: an opening, a spiritual experience, a sense of peace and inner happiness.

Thus to really touch we need to stay very mindful and focused, not distracted by past, present and future, to help us to embody this state of mind so that we can touch in the right way. And by having an open spacious mindset our energy starts to flow freely through our whole being, which will result in a touch full of love, compassion and inner bliss and joy.

Chapter 14:

Okuden Reiki II

*If you search for your true self outwardly, with your ordinary,
dualistic human consciousness, you will never find it.*
– *The Light That Shines Through Infinity by Dainin Katagiri*

Okuden means inner or hidden teachings, which relates to
going inwards and finding what is hidden inside of ourselves:
emptiness, non-duality, our great bright light or whatever we
name it. Our essence. Hence do not look outwards to find
it, it is right there already inside of us. This is also why we
need to internalize the practices taught within Okuden. They
are like keys to unlock what has been hidden inside of us.
Do not get distracted by the keys themselves. If we hold a
key in our hand and have endless discussions about what it
looks like, or compare our keys with others, then we never
use the key. And therefore we never will open that door to
our True Self. Sit and internalize the key; open your mind
with it. This is why Mikao Usui called this level Okuden, a
big pointer to internalization. Do not throw away the keys
too early. We might have a glimpse of our True Self, think we
have "gotten it" and stop using the key. But we forget that
the winds of our habitual patterns are strong and will blow
the door closed, until we open it again. And then sometimes
we think or pretend that we are still in touch with our True
Self. So keep checking, keep practicing with the keys until the
door stays open 24 hours a day. And even then, we have to
keep practicing.

In this book, I have only included the most important
elements of Okuden. There are other basic practices like byosen
reikan ho and reiji-ho, but these are just there to help you to

become more flowing, more intuitive with hands on/off healing. Very good practices, but not the most important.

The most basic technique in Dento Reiki [Usui Reiki Ryôhô Gakkai] involves detecting a Byosen and then placing the hands on the affected area in order to perform an effective healing treatment... Different Reiki healers experience different kinds of sensations.
– A Modern Reiki Method for Healing By Hiroshi Doi

Hatsurei-ho

The first practice of Okuden is hatsurei-ho, which is a combination of three practices taught in Shoden Reiki I. Within the Japanese esoteric tradition, it is very common to first learn individual practices and later on when the student has gotten the hang of these practices, laid a kind of base, to put them together into one single practice.

Hatsu 発 means to arise, to give birth, to reveal what is hidden or to emit.
Rei 霊 means spirit, soul or inconceivable spiritual ability.
Ho 法 means dharma, ultimate truth or method.

We therefore could say that hatsurei-ho means, "a method to reveal our hidden inconceivable spiritual ability." What is this hidden inconceivable spiritual ability? It is emptiness, non-duality, great bright light, our True Self. This also means that we need to keep practicing this method, not just once or twice, but until we have laid bare our True Self. And even then we have to keep practicing it. Imagine you have a diamond, pure and shiny. If you leave it out in the world it will get dusty, so you have to keep polishing it to maintain its brilliance. It is the same with our True Self.

That energy gives forth its own light, shining from your whole body, which others can see.

– The Light That Shines Through Infinity by Dainin Katagiri

This is an essential practice that was also being taught nearly a hundred years ago by Kaiji Tomita, a student of Mikao Usui. We can find this in Kaiji Tomita's book, *Reiki To Jinjutsu – Tomita Ryu Téaté Ryôhô*, published in 1933. Fumio Ogawa (1906-1998?) wrote a booklet, *Everyone can do Reiki*, in which we also find hatsurei-ho; in fact he links it with the teachings of Zen Master Hakuin Ekaku. And we also can find hatsurei-ho within the *Reiki Ryôhô no Shiori*, which is a booklet handed out by the Usui Reiki Ryôhô Gakkai. Thus we can see how important it is. The deeper we go within Mikao Usui's teachings the more we start to see that hands on/off healing is only a very small part, and that the essential teachings are all about rediscovering our hidden inconceivable spiritual ability.

So let's practice hatsurei-ho as much as we can, preferably daily, so that we can create heaven on earth: a world in which we all have laid bare our True Self, pure compassion and wisdom.

Practicing hatsurei-ho:

Step 1 (kenyokū hō)

Again, don't forget to use all the preparation practices. We do this with any practice we do, so often that it becomes us, in all we do.

1. Gassho – to center the mind and set intent while standing or sitting.

2a. Place your right hand on the left shoulder. Breathe into the hara, and on the out-breath, sweep diagonally down from the left shoulder to the right hip.

2b. On the in-breath into the hara, place your left hand on the right shoulder and, on the out-breath, sweep down diagonally from right shoulder to left hip.

2c. Breathe into the hara, returning your right hand to the left shoulder and, on the out-breath, sweep diagonally down from left shoulder to right hip.

3a. On the next in-breath into the hara, place your right hand on the left shoulder; on the out-breath, sweep downward along the arm to the fingertips, palm facing upwards.

3b. On the next in-breath into the hara, place your left hand on the right shoulder; on the out-breath, sweep downward along the arm to the fingertips, palm facing upwards.

3c. On the next in-breath into the hara, place your right hand on the left shoulder; on the out-breath, sweep downward along the arm to the fingertips, palm facing upwards. Move on to step 2.

Step 2 (jōshin kokyū hō)

1. Sit and gassho.

2. Place your hands in your lap, palms facing upwards.

3. With each in-breath, feel/visualize a bright energy coming in through the nose and bring it down to the hara, just below your navel. When you do this, link the visual with the breath and the mind.

4. Feel/visualize the bright energy, the breath and the mind expanding through your body.

5. On the out-breath, expand the bright energy, the breath and the mind out of the body, through your skin, out into infinity.

6. Repeat steps 3 to 5 for 10 minutes, and then move on to the next step.

Step 3 (seishin toitsu)

1. With your hands in the gassho position, focus on your hara. On the in-breath, begin to bring the energy/breath and mind into your fingertips – hands. Feel the energy/ breath and mind move through your arms, down through

your body and into the hara.

2. On the out-breath, visualize energy/breath and mind moving from the hara back up through the body and then to the arms and out through the hands – fingertips.

3. Do this for 10 minutes.

Step 4 (no-form)

1. Just sit in that space of no-form, but be aware with clarity if you are getting distracted by past, present, and future. Then either readjust your focus on that empty state, or if that is not possible, do any of the previous steps again.

Through practicing this meditation method we start to calm the mind; the energy will therefore nurture the body to help the body stay healthy. This is important if we want to help others, as we cannot help others if we do not feel well within our own mind and body. Through this practice our breathing slows down, which in turn can have a positive effect on many things within our mind and body: heart rate, blood pressure, or anxiety, for example.

> *The ordinary person's rate of breathing is said to be 18 times per minute. As for those of us who breathe with the tanden [hara], the frequency of our breathing ranges from two or three to five or six times per minute. In the beginning it cannot be done without conscious effort.*
> *– Introduction to Zen Training: A Physical Approach to Meditation and Mind-Body Training by Omori Sogen*

As Zen Master Omori Sogen points out, this slowing down cannot be done without conscious effort, samatha, focus. But make sure the focus is not too tight or too loose, just perfect like a guitar string. Through this focus and specific breathing practice, we start to stimulate the hara, that inner fire.

When ki 氣 is pure and uncontaminated there is no illness. When the ki of a human being is orderly this ki will circulate throughout the entire body. When the ki is not orderly, here and there this ki will stagnate.

– Kottō-roku 骨董録 Record of Curios, Zen master Takuan Sōhō 澤菴 宗彭 (1573-1645)

Our mind/ki will be uncontaminated because we are focusing; we are not contaminating it with worry, anger, or not being grateful. We are not being distracted by the past, present, future. Thus our mind/ki stays orderly, and therefore it will start to circulate through our whole body. This is why it is so important to practice this method, not just once in a while but daily, ideally for at least 20 to 40 minutes, so that our mind/ki will not stagnate. Stagnation keeps us stuck and can create all sorts of issues, as well as hindering our practice, our progress, spiritual growth and development.

First Symbol and Mantra

This is how I explain the mudra, but immediately you ask, "Oh, what is that?" And then you want to discuss it, but there is no solution to your confusion. Finally I have to say, "Please keep your mouth shut, and just do this simple practice. If you are interested in this mudra, you can study later. You can find it explained in a big book." Still, no matter how long you study the mudra intellectually, it is nothing but a symbol. But actually that symbol is not merely a symbol. Through your practice you can really know the meaning of this mudra.

– The Light That Shines Through Infinity by Dainin Katagiri

In this book, I show the kanji for each symbol, but I do not include the symbols themselves, or the method for drawing them. It's best to learn this from a qualified teacher who guides you into the practice in a proper way. But I will describe why the symbols are there and how you can use them to take your practice a step deeper. Again symbols and mantras are keys, so work with them or you will never open that door. Again, which door? The door to our True Self. To practice perfectly, we need to know why the symbols and mantras are there, what they point towards, and how to use them in the proper way. We can practice in all sorts of ways but if we do not practice in the way it was intended, we might have not the right outcome, remembering our True Self.

So, why are the symbols and mantras there in Okuden Reiki II? They are a samatha practice, to help us to calm the mind through focus; in this case we focus on a symbol and/or a mantra. Without this supreme focus, we cannot enter vipassana, which is symbolized by the Shinpiden Reiki III symbol and mantra dai kômyô 大光明.

When mind reaches a state of complete stillness, its profound nature can be revealed. Stillness of mind corresponds to samatha, and the experience of mind's nature to vipasyana.
– Luminous Mind by Kalu Rinpoche

Thus only through complete stillness of mind can our profound nature dai kômyô 大光明 be revealed. Hence when we move through the system of Reiki too quickly, we will not get the full benefit of Mikao Usui's teachings; we are not laying bare our True Self. We also lose the full benefit when we use the symbols and mantras externally, because when we do not use them internally, our mind will not be completely still. In fact, the more we use them externally, the busier our mind becomes; so we are kind of agitating the already agitated mind. Why? Because when we use the symbols externally we use them for dual concepts, for aspects of the past, present, and future.

The first symbol and mantra are two separate tools; the

mantra is not the name of the symbol. They can be used together or separately, however, depending on whether we need more focus, more pegs so to speak. Imagine a tent: when there is no wind at all we can just place the tent on the ground, no pegs are needed. When times are easy and our mind is calm, maybe we can just work with our breath to stay focused. But when there is a bit of wind coming up, we need a few pegs to hold the tent in place. The tent is like our mind which gets bowled over by the wind. In times like these, we can use a mantra or a symbol to help us focus. But when the wind becomes stronger and stronger, we need more pegs, we need sanmitsu, we need to really engage our mind, body, and speech, hence we need the body – right position, the mind – a symbol, and speech – a mantra.

The first mantra is Choku Rei 直霊 and it translates as straight spirit or direct spirit. This comes from old Shintoism, and sometimes is also pronounced as Naohi.

The term chokurei 直霊. Choku (直) means "direct" and rei (霊) means "spirit". Chokurei is the light emanating directly from God to from the origin of humanity. Chokurei could be translated as "God in the human world," "Direct Spirit," or "Divine Self."
– God and Man: Guideposts for Spiritual Peace and Awakening by Masahisa Goi (1916-1980)

Thus this mantra is about remembering our divine self, our essence. And what is this essence? Non-duality – emptiness, again and again Mikao Usui is pointing out the same thing; why? Because we can be so stubborn, so blind that even if we practice the system of Reiki for many years and claim to have mastered it, often we still do not see what Mikao Usui is pointing out. Hence we have to chant this mantra internally to reawaken our divine self. If we use the mantra externally, our divine self will not be laid bare because our divine self is not external to us. It is not outside of us; it is right here, inside of us. It is not something we have to accumulate through our practice. No, the practice is there to realize that we are our divine self, right at this moment in time. Right here today.

There I encountered my own divine spirit [Choku Rei 直霊].
– From Living Like the Blue Sky: five talks by Masahisa Goi

That we have to realize we are a divine spirit in this body is not only pointed out with this mantra, but also within the first symbol. The first symbol has its roots in the ancient kanji of kami 神. Some years ago when I practiced Shugendo in Japan on Mt. Omine, I spoke to the residing priest there, Kyosei Yamauchi Sensei. I drew for him the first symbol as we use it within the system of Reiki. I was not even finished when he exclaimed, "That means go to kami." This of course makes perfect sense as the word kami is often translated as god or divine being. Hence when we internalize the first symbol we are going to our kami, we are going back to our divine spirit. Thus when we see the original Japanese meaning of the first symbol and mantra, we realize that they both point to our divine self, and that we do not need to look for our divine self externally but internally. Hence we need to meditate on the symbol and chant the mantra. A good Reiki teacher, preferably one who has internalized this themselves, can help you with it, as this really needs to be taught in person!

Let's recap this, so that we gain a good understanding as to why Mikao Usui placed this symbol and mantra within his teachings. First, the symbols and mantras are a samatha practice, to help us to focus. We have to focus, letting go of our distractions, past, present, and future, else we cannot lay bare our divine self. The symbols and mantras have to be internalized; they are keys, so that we can remember that hidden inside is our True Self. They are not magical symbols and mantras which we wave around or speak. This is easy to see; if they were then we could use them once and presto – we are in the state of our divine self. But let's be honest; it doesn't work that way.

Because if we are really in that state of our divine self, then we would have no more anger and worry, we would be grateful for whatever comes our way, we would be true to our way and our being and we would be emanating a compassion which does not change due to circumstances. Thus, now we start to realize that the symbol and mantra are all about laying bare the precepts. So check within yourself; don't fool yourself or be fooled. This is why we work to have perfect practice, else our practice will not bear the right fruit. And instead of having the fruit of emptiness, our great bright light, we have the fruit of duality, confusion, ego – me, me, me – and a kindness which changes upon the circumstances... this in itself is not compassionate, to ourselves or to the world.

Second Symbol and Mantra

We need to understand why we are practicing; we can know the practice but if we do not know why we are practicing, then we are a bit lost. Within the precepts, Mikao Usui used the phrase, The spiritual medicine of 10.000 illnesses. So we need to know why we take the medicine, right? Just taking medicine without knowing why would be like being healthy and starting to take some kind of medicine that only might trigger problems. So it is very important to know why we practice and what the aim is. Why do we use a visualization? Why do we use a mantra? These are very important elements because through this we create clarity in our practice.

The second symbol and mantra are two separate elements, the mantra in this case, is also not the name for the symbol. Again we can use either the symbol or the mantra separately or together depending on the state of our mind; if the wind blowing is strong, then we can use both. If we feel too distracted by the past, present, future and we can't seem to focus, then it is very important to use more pegs to secure the tent of our mind. Because if we are not focused, then we are just practicing distraction during our visualization or chanting of the mantra. If we are mindlessly chanting by rote, this only results in pain in our throat and not in laying bare our True Self. Because for that to happen we need to stay focused, samatha practice.

The second mantra is sei heki 性癖.

Sei 性 nature – inner essence – innate
Heki 癖 disposition – mannerism – habit

A primary dictionary definition of disposition is "a person's inherent qualities of mind and character." We thus can translate sei heki as "natural disposition" or "a person's natural innate inherent quality of mind and character". So when we look at sei heki, our natural disposition, what is this natural quality of mind? This natural quality of our mind is emptiness, non-duality. Again Mikao Usui points out emptiness, compassion, and non-duality. Why? Because it is the natural inherent quality of our mind; this is really what he was teaching. Far more than just hands on/off healing, he was teaching a profound method for self-illumination.

> When ki follows this guideline it becomes straight and proper. When it does not it becomes crooked. Inside humans and objects this guideline or principle is also known as "nature" (sei 性). When nature is activated it is called the great mind/heart, the mind/heart of the Way, or straight mind. Conversely, what turns against nature is called the deluded mind. The point that Takuan is trying to make, of course, is that the mind/heart should try to follow the guideline, that is, the Way. This is how everything becomes peaceful.
> – Juhn Y. Ahn, Worms, Germs, and Technologies of the Self – Religion, Sword Fighting, and Medicine in Early Modern Japan

As you can see in the above quote, Zen Master Takuan Sōhō (1573-1645) also pointed to our nature, sei 性, and that it is inside of us, our inner guideline or principle. Therefore we have to internalize the mantra through chanting it the right way. Not just mindlessly but with supreme focus, non-distraction, deep from within the hara. When we chant and we breathe deeply into the hara with pure focus, the practice becomes like a magnifying glass, igniting the inner fire. This fire is needed for the mist and rain to rise and fall which in turn is needed for our direct experience of our True Self. This is the inner workings of nature, of our human nature, as we are made out of the same elements of nature itself; we are nature. A well-known Japanese Zen master states, *"Sei heki is not about explanation, all understanding needs to be let go of, and there you find zen."* Zen is the same as sei heki; it is our essence, it is who we truly are. All the masters of old pointed towards the same but we seem to get so distracted by the different words, symbols, mantras, techniques, that we forget where we are aiming it. It is like a signpost; we are not following the signposts at all these days. Instead we grab hold of the signpost and start to intellectualize it, we compare it with other signposts, and we are so busy doing that that we completely miss the point of why we practice.

The natural disposition of emptiness arises as great compassion and you enter into unbiased compassionate love.
– Khenchen Palden Sherab Rinpoche

Through practicing the mantra in the right way we will lay bare great compassion, and unbiased love, which does not change depending on the situation. Mikao Usui also pointed this out within the precepts, and the mantras are all about the embodiment of the precepts in every action we take in our daily life.

The second symbol has its heritage in the bonji of hrih or

kiriiku which is the seed syllable of Amitabha Buddha. A seed syllable is the supreme condensation of the ultimate truth. Amitabha or Amida means infinite light; hence the deity is a personification of the ultimate truth, infinite light. Thus again Mikao Usui points towards emptiness because this infinite light has no beginning and end, and we cannot grab hold of light. This light is the light – energy – which emanates from emptiness. We have to realize that we are none other than this infinite light, and to do this we have to internalize the symbol. But what does this mean, internalize; that you become the symbol? Or is there a deeper meaning to this? First of all, if we see it as something dual – this is me and this is the symbol – then we are still working dualistically. In fact, internalization is a dissolution. If we use the imagery of a raindrop which represents the symbol, entering a lake which represents ourselves, now we cannot distinguish one from the other: the raindrop and the lake, the symbol and ourselves. This is the embodiment of the symbol: non-duality. When this happens through prolonged dedicated meditation practice, we realize that we are this infinite light, no beginning and end.

Now imagine a thought arising within this infinite light; light is not sticky, so the thought doesn't stick. Light does not cling either, so what happens to the thought? It just dissolves, light into light. Hence when we have laid bare this infinite light of compassion and wisdom, nothing sticks. And when the thoughts don't stick there will be no anger or worry. There will just be compassion, a compassion which does not change depending on our moods or circumstance, because this compassion is light, is emptiness, is infinite. Again, this doesn't mean that we become a zombie, or an empty-headed shell with no thoughts. It means that we can see our thoughts with clarity, without clinging to them.

We can use this symbol very superficially, draw it here and there, but that does not have much use. If that was the case we could draw this symbol on each person we see and presto – there will be no more anger and worry within that person. But we all know that this is not really how it works. This is why to really get the most out of Mikao Usui's teachings we have to sit in meditation and meditate with this symbol, so that over time we can lay bare this infinite light. When we have laid bare our infinite light, our True Self, we have cut the root of all our problems; why? Because the thoughts don't stick anymore, they come and just dissolve again within the infinite light.

Third Symbol and Mantra

If you practice mindfulness based on dualistic understanding, you will never have a peaceful mind.
– The Light That Shines Through Infinity by Dainin Katagiri

The third symbol and mantra are a bit different; in this case, the symbol is really the kanji of the mantra. Thus we can see that the first two symbols and mantras are really a symbol and a separate mantra, and in this case we can see that the mantra is the direct translation of the kanji/symbol. The kanji is compressed, with the individual characters close together, which was done to make it more "secret", so to speak. This was not an unusual practice in the Japanese esoteric traditions. But what does this kanji stand for?

The right mind operates at each time and in each place to make you take the right attitude and act properly without deviating from the Way.
– Master Sogaku

Hon Sha Ze Sho Nen 本者是正念.
Hon 本 means true, book, origin, real, to find the origin in. In Buddhist tradition, Hon is often used in combination with other

kanji to point to our original self or True Self. For example, honshin means true mind or original mind.

Sha 者 means a person, someone, the one [who, which], he/she who is.

Ze 是 means right, correct, just so, this, justice, perfectly, it is this.

Sho 正 means right, correct, true, straight, the basis of correct knowledge, righteous.

Nen 念 means thought, feeling, mindfulness, mind, memory, meditative wisdom, patience, forbearance.

Shonen 正念 is part of the Buddha's teachings of the Eightfold Noble Path, which stands for "right mindfulness". Right mindfulness means to stay in that mindful state continuously, or in other words, to rest in our natural mind all the time, the natural mind of our True Self, emptiness.

The direct translation of this phrase is: "My original nature is a right thought." It also can be translated as "My original nature is right mind," "My original nature is right mindfulness," or in a more direct way we can say, "I am right mind." In the case of "I am right mind," the "I" is not the ego "I" but the "I" of the True Self. When we rediscover our True Self there is still a person there, so we still have to say, for example, "I am drinking a coffee." A person who has rediscovered their True Self will not cling to this "I", while a person who has not rediscovered their True Self will. But what is this Right Mind, this Right Thought? Right, as in the Japanese esoteric tradition, points out our non-dual nature, emptiness.

The No-Mind is the same as the Right Mind. It neither congeals nor fixes itself in one place. It is called No-Mind when the mind has neither discrimination nor thought but wanders about the entire body and extends throughout the entire self.
– The Unfettered Mind by Takuan Sōhō

Zen Master Takuan Sōhō points it out beautifully; it is a mind that has not fixed itself in one place, in past, present, or future. This mind is thus wide open; it can wander freely through our whole body and the entire universe, our True Self. This mind does not get stuck with anger and worry, and this mind is our true mind, our essence. Hence we can see that Mikao Usui again pointed out our True Self: emptiness, non-duality.

Human consciousness can go anywhere in the universe in an instant. You must endeavor to develop your consciousness quickly and not to rely on the symbols for too long.

– note from a student of Mikao Usui

So we must not use the symbol for too long, but that doesn't mean we have to stop using it and think we have understood. We can only stop using it when we have developed the consciousness of emptiness. Why can the human consciousness go anywhere in the universe in an instant? Because of its non-dual nature. This also gives a hint about "distance healing" – in an instant. This means there is no distance to be covered, because the consciousness is already instantaneously here.

Therefore this symbol and mantra is not there for "distance healing." It is there for ourselves, to lay bare our right mind, the mind of non-duality, of emptiness. Again and again Mikao Usui points to the same thing, and yet somehow we don't see it. Thus if we want to practice Mikao Usui's teachings, we have to aim for what he is pointing at, the laying bare of our True Self, emptiness, compassion, non-duality. This means again that we have to let go of dual concepts in our practice, the concept of I am here and you are there. We let go of the concept of this Reiki is different from that, this is a higher vibration than that, Reiki is there and I am here, now Reiki is on and now Reiki is off. These are all dualistic ideas and therefore not really promoting a deep understanding of non-duality. If we practice this way, our aim is duality and not non-duality. And if our aim is duality then we will always be in conflict. Always there will be anger and worry and fear around the corner, and we will never have a peaceful mind, let alone a peaceful world. Normally we live in a dual world with a dual mind, but we have to learn how to live in our dual world with the mind of non-duality.

When we see dualistically we are insecure and unbalanced.
– Ten Ox Herding Pictures by Zen Master Shodo Harada

Thus if we promote duality in our practice and/or teachings, we promote insecurity and being unbalanced. And that is not what a spiritual practice is about. A spiritual practice is about promoting compassion, wisdom, and pure love – not insecurity. Please contemplate this: what is your aim, insecurity and feeling unbalanced? Or do you want your aim to be that you feel secure and balanced? It is only ourselves who can make that choice. But we have to aim correctly, else we will never hit the right target and the world will stay in turmoil. Thus if we say we want the world to be a better place and at the same time we fill our teachings and practice with dual concepts, then there is an issue: they contradict each other. This is why we have to make sure our teachings come from the right place, a direct experience of emptiness, and that we practice in the right way.

In Sanskrit, the word for "right" is samma. It means "to go along with," "to go together," "to turn together." It originally comes from a term that means "to unite." So "right" is a state of being in which everything can live together, or turn together, united. Right is a state of human life in which we live in peace and harmony with all other beings. It is right, beyond our ideas of right or wrong, good or bad.
– You Have to Say Something: Manifesting Zen Insight by Dainin Katagiri

So please contemplate Mikao Usui's teachings carefully; we have to contemplate our practice so that we practice correctly, practice right, for the sake of the world. This is true compassion. We can get caught up in what lineage we practice, we can get caught up in which tradition we practice, or we can just practice the right way in which we realize our right mind, our True Self.

We cannot have a healed society, we cannot have change, we cannot have justice, if we do not reclaim and repair the human spirit.
— Angel Kyodo Williams

Kototama

The way we work with the mantras of the system of Reiki is Kototama; we chant them in a specific way. This again cannot be taught in a book and needs to be experienced and taught by a good Reiki teacher who has had many direct experiences through this chanting. For example, when I was with a group of students in Japan in 2019, we met with my teacher Takeda Hakusai Ajari, and he had us chant a specific sound a few times, one by one. He observed the student who was chanting to see if they were chanting from their hara and also to see/feel how their mind, body, speech was during it. Through this direct experience, Takeda Ajari knew how each person's practice is and how their state of mind is and how their health is.

The kototama is not a theory or even a teaching. It's the life energy, or ki, that gives birth to consciousness in all its myriad forms.
— Aikido and Words of Power: The Sacred Sounds of Kototama by William Gleason

Kototama has a long history in Japan and started to gain popularity again in Mikao Usui's time; this was also due to the fact that the Meiji Emperor and his wife were modern kototama researchers and practitioners. The word kototama 言霊 literally means "word spirit" or "soul". But it also stands for the spiritual (tama) power of sound (koto). Within kototama there are mother and father sounds. The mother sounds are the vowels, which are the most important; the father sounds are the consonants. When the mother and father sounds are united, they create child sounds. There are 5 mother sounds, 8 father sounds, 5 half mother sounds and 32 child sounds. The 5 mother sounds also interlink with the 5 elements of earth, water, fire, air, and space.

The sounds are chanted in specific patterns to trigger very precise states of mind, which we might also experience on an energetic level, as both mind and energy are intertwined. And this has an effect on our body, thus we need to chant from that state of mind of sanmitsu. The ultimate aim of chanting these kototama is to realize our interconnectedness with the universe. The more we start to realize this interconnectedness, the more we experience that everything is kototama. And when chanting from this perspective of emptiness, non-duality, then it is not us who is chanting kototama; it is the whole universe that is chanting.

> *Finally we did the "deep chant", taking the vowels a, i, u, e, o and energetically singing them out with our whole body and soul, sound by sound, as u, a, i, e... Sensei always said, "teaching this discipline is the greatest kindness. The first step in your practice is to practice this."*
> – *Journey in Search of the Way by Satomi Myodo (1896-1978)*

Satomi Myodo learned this in the time that Mikao Usui was alive and teaching. It was a common practice in the esoteric traditions, and within Zen.

Why is chanting kototama so important? Because of sanmitsu. Remember, body is very physical: we can touch it, feel it, see it. However, mind is very subtle; we can't touch it, or feel it, or see it. While speech is in between body and mind, we can feel it and hear it. Yet speech is not as physical as the body and not as subtle as the mind. To work with our very subtle mind is difficult for most of us. Hence speech or chanting is a bridge between body and mind. It takes the practice from gross (body) to subtle (speech) to very subtle (mind). This is why we first have hands on healing within the system of Reiki, in Shoden Reiki I, and it is only in Okuden Reiki II that we move to a more subtle practice. It is much easier to first practice with the body because it is so tangible, all the old teachings work in the same way. Thus within the system of Reiki we progress from body teachings and practices, to speech teaching and practices, so that finally we can work with mind teachings and practices, because the mind is the most subtle of all. Of course this doesn't take place overnight and this is why kototama needs to be chanted over and over and over again, so that we get the direct experience of what kototama really represents.

Hara is not only the physical center of the body; properly understood, it is also the center of our spiritual energy.
– The Spiritual Foundations of Aikido by William Gleason

One of the key elements to remember when chanting kototama is that the sound needs to come from our lower abdomen, the hara or tanden. When the sound comes from the hara, we perform deep breathing (Okinagaho in Shintoism). Through this kind of deep breathing the sounds can resonate through our whole physical being, due to our mind being calm and centered. Imagine a singing bowl: if the bowl is upside down it doesn't resonate; it needs to be placed the right way up. This is what we do when we focus on the hara, else we are chanting from our head which is like the singing bowl being upside down. Now imagine that you put lots of stuff in the singing bowl (turned right way up) and then strike it. Can it still resonate? No, it can't, as it is full of stuff! So for kototama to really resonate through our whole being, we need to be like the singing bowl: empty. Our mind needs to be empty; this is why we always have to work with emptiness again and again and again until we begin to experience it. So again we can ask ourselves, empty of what? Empty of holding on to the past, present, and future. This can be a challenge. But thus the more we chant kototama and the more we start to breathe deeply into our hara, the more empty our mind will be and the more the sound will vibrate through our whole being. And ultimately, the more we will start to realize our True Self, our empty nature, our non-dual state of mind.

The kototama is not merely the sound of the human voice. It is the red blood in your hara, boiling over with life. When I chant the sounds of A O U E I, the gods which perform the functions of these kototama gather around me. A true human being can do this and a great deal more.

– Morihei Ueshiba, The Spiritual Foundations of Aikido by William Gleason

Each specific sound also has different meanings. Let's look at the first kototama within the system of Reiki, Choku Rei: OUEI.

O = Water – continuation of a spiritual action – rushing stream – moving down – physical health – connection – accumulation – understanding – sinking
U = Unity – universal body/spirit – returns to itself – originates deep in the belly – pure existence – void (form is emptiness and emptiness is form – Heart Sutra) – direct spirit – balance
E = Fire – expanding – branches out to become the channels in the body – seeking – spiritual growth – rising
I = Earth – center – one point – life force – will of life – senses – control center/grounding – power – perception – vitality – stability – expanding outside of the body

The U dimension is the simultaneous reality of gross matter and pure spirit as one and the same energy. It is the absolute basis of reality and it is our spirit, naobi [naobi is the same kanji as choku rei], at one with that of the universe.
— The Spiritual Foundations of Aikido by William Gleason

William Gleason points out that choku rei – naobi – naohi, is the embodiment of pure spirit in our physical body and is linked to the U dimension. Thus if we look deeply into this kototama, we can see that it helps us to become grounded (water always flows down) and centered in our body. And from this grounded and centered state, we can expand up and outwards. This is why Mikao Usui taught OUEI as the first kototama, as we first need to become aware of our physical being before we can experience this expansion up and outwards. It is in this physical being that we need to embody the universe; this is the body. When we look closely we also see water and fire, which of course we also see in the kanji of Reiki, in the fire rising upwards and the water raining down. All of Mikao Usui's teachings are interconnected; not one element is a standalone element. Therefore we need to practice in the right way to create the right foundation and therefore we reach the right destination.

If you try to fill your life just from the top, by gaining knowledge, then your head is very big. But the knowledge you gain is hard to carry because it's pretty heavy. It makes your head spin, and it's easy to lose your balance.
— The Light That Shines Through Infinity by Dainin Katagiri

Our practice is like filling a vessel; when we pour something in the vessel it goes straight to the bottom and then it slowly rises until the vessel is filled. We cannot start filling it from the top. But this is what we do when we breathe wrongly, high up in the chest; we only fill the top of the lungs. And this is not natural;

this triggers anger, worry, and fear. Thus we need to start with the direct experience in our hara, filling up our body the right way, so to speak. This is also why it is better not to get too intellectual about these practices and sounds.

Within the various sects of both Shinto and Buddhism, the classification of elements is not consistent; it changes with the view being expressed and sometimes it depends on the physical experience of the practitioner.

Aikido and Words of Power: The Sacred Sounds of Kototama by William Gleason

Don't get too confused by the intellectual side of it all. This is why traditionally the teacher would not really explain all of this, so that the student could first of all have the direct experience and not be in their head. We can always intellectualize too much, but we can never practice enough.

The second kototama is Sei Heki: EI E KI.

E = Fire – evaluation of our spiritual practice – seeking – creation – pursuit – branching out – courage – clear judgement/ wisdom – non-doing – spiritual growth – intellectual – rising
I = Will of life – power of life – center – senses – life force – earth – power – perception – vitality – stability
E = Fire – evaluation of our spiritual practice – seeking – creation – pursuit – branching out – courage – clear judgement/ wisdom – non-doing – spiritual growth – intellectual – rising
KI = Light of fire – fullness of our will of life – foundation of life energy, breath, intention – tying Ki together – releasing tension – manifestation of nature – source of the relative world – true will – intention – thunder – engages the wheels of creation – cutting through all obstructions like a sword

As we can now see there is lots of fire within this kototama. This is why we first have to work with the first kototama OUEI, to create a stable base else the fire will rise in our body and this will only trigger more anger and worry. Here we can clearly see that the right foundation and the right time of practice is important. Again a good Reiki teacher will be able to show and teach you these important elements. This is why we would first chant the first kototama for maybe a year on a daily basis, ideally 45 minutes each session and always in a focused way, samatha, not just chanting mindlessly. And this is why the kototama also needs to be directed inwards; in doing this we can stimulate our internal energy, so that it can follow the pattern of nature, rain, mist, fire, the natural cycles.

At the time of uttering the syllables EI, KEI and KI he makes the mudra of beckoning the fire God, by bending the index finger. The flame of the fire is considered as the Fire god himself.
– Buddhist Fire Ritual in Japan by Musashi Tachikawa

The third kototama is Hon Sha Ze Sho Nen: O A ZE O NE.

O = Continuation of a spiritual action – rushing stream – moving down – water – self organization – connection – accumulation – physical health – understanding – sinking (hO) expansion of light opening wider – physicalized form – spiritual origin blazing forth – ripening of spirit
A = Spiritual action – unborn – space
ZE = Evaluation of our spiritual practice (sometimes also seen as SE). There are the "pure" or "base" syllables. Some of them have voiced counterparts ("ka-ga, to-do, sa-za", etc.)
... SE = Fire within water – all light and action through the center bound together – concentration of the five senses.
O = Continuation of a spiritual action – rushing stream – moving down – water – self-organization – connection – accumulation – physical health – understanding – sinking

(hO) expansion of light opening wider – physicalized form
– Spiritual origin blazing forth – ripening of spirit
NE = Letting go of judgement – non grasping – Fire/water
ki – the root of intellect

Here again we can see that it comes from our physical body –
physicalized form – and that we have to work with the body,
because the body is the vehicle for our mind. Shinshin kaizen, as
Mikao Usui pointed out within his precepts, is such an important
teaching. And again we can see the concept of fire and water. This
again is pointing to the inner workings of the kanji of Reiki and
the inner workings of our own energy system. Plus we have to
let go of judgement, grasping, as it is through this that our light
can start to blaze forward. Remember the practice of hatsurei-
ho, emanating a greater amount of spirit? This is pointing out
the same thing. Through looking deeper into these teachings we
start to see that all the practices taught within the system of Reiki
are pointing to the same aim, our great bright light, the great
bright light of emptiness and non-duality, the great bright light
of compassion and wisdom. This is why each kototama has to
be practiced individually over a prolonged time, first maybe a
year or maybe two years the first kototama, then the second, also
for a year or two. Now we are creating the right foundation and
environment to work with the third kototama, so that we can
have that direct experience of non-duality, right mind.

Distance Healing

By now we might understand that there is no distance at
all. This is what Mikao Usui was pointing out; everything is
interconnected.

Everything in the Universe possesses Reiki without any exception.
– note from a student of Mikao Usui

With each practice, no matter if we look at the precepts, the breath meditations, hands on/off healing, the symbols and mantras and also the reiju, Mikao Usui points towards non-duality, that everything is Reiki without exception. Thus what is there to "send"? This means that during a "distance healing" we are not really sending anything at all. But what do we have to do then? We have to sit in meditation, and remember that interconnectedness, this non-dual right mind. And in that state of mind, the other person will take whatever they need. And then something interesting happens. When we sit in that state of mind of interconnectedness we realize that the whole universe will benefit from that session, because we are the universe and the universe is us. As the *Reiki Ryôhô no Shiori* booklet published by the Usui Reiki Ryôhô states, "Strict teachings and rules of Master Usui: One of the most strict rules which he taught us is that your spirit as a small universe has to be always united with the spiritual power of the whole universe as one."

As we have seen, one of the translations of hon sha ze sho nen is, "my original nature is right mindfulness." Here Mikao Usui pointed to that deep interconnectedness within our mind.

Your unified mind is lots of mind, collected as one. This is called mind-full-ness.
– The Light That Shines Through Infinity by Dainin Katagiri

Being in that state of right mindfulness we start to realize the deep interconnectedness with all that is. That all our minds are collected as one, non-duality. Therefore there is no need to connect to anybody or anything; we are all interconnected already, our minds collected as one. This is real mindfulness. This is what we have to remember.

Many people say, "I need to connect to my friend who needs healing," or when we perform hands on/healing we might say, "I need to connect to the person on the table." Or we say, "I will send energy," or "Please send me energy." But this really indicates that you are feeling disconnected. There is nothing to connect to in the first place as by nature we are already interconnected. We can never separate ourselves from anything; we cannot step out of the universe for a bit and then reenter it – impossible. Hence we also have to check our speech, remember sanmitsu – mind, body, speech. Our speech indicates how our mind is thinking. So if we say we think we are Being Reiki or think we are in that non-dual state of mind and yet our speech is all about connecting, duality, then there is a contradiction happening. Thus our speech is really showing that we have not integrated non-duality in our mind, that it is just an intellectual concept and hasn't yet soaked into our mind, body, and speech, like the mist which soaks our whole being. This is why we need to have clarity within our mind, so that our practice is clear and that our aim is direct.

But here is a tricky part: of course we can still call it "distance healing" as long as we know that there is no distance at all, that it all takes place in our own mind. So if we hear someone or ourselves saying, "distance healing," are they/we saying it for the sake of convenience or someone else's understanding, or out of habit? And, most importantly, is their/our mind in reality resting in that non-dual state? Or are they/we saying it and their/our mind is still getting caught up in duality? This is not easy to check and therefore we need this clarity of the great bright light, so that we can see things clearly. If we have a very bright light we see things very clearly, things we might not see when we are in the dark. The brighter the light is, the further we can see into the distance, far enough to see that there really is no distance at all.

We always have our own mind with us and therefore we also do not need any external prop to perform "distance healing". But this "distance healing" in an interconnected state of mind might not be so easy; this is why Mikao Usui only taught it at the end of

Okuden Reiki II. If we still have lots of fears and worries, we might feel that this interconnectedness is scary, we might have the idea that we pick something up from the other person. But again, as we have discussed earlier, this comes from the false sense of the "I". This is why Mikao Usui pointed out again and again, initially in Shoden Reiki I and in the first stages of Okuden Reiki II, that we have to let go of this "I". And only then can we perform the deeper layers of "distance healing". Remember, this interconnectedness is like a raindrop dissolving into a lake or a cup of water, there is now no distinction between the two, impossible to detect which one is which. Therefore "distance healing" is also not sharing space; sharing space means one person gets half of the space that the other person has, and again, this is not the right way to see it.

But this individual self that I recognize is not my real existence; it is only something temporarily running through my conscious mind in the realm of time. The original, pure nature of my existence is the realm of space. In the realm of space, things are not separate and independent; all beings are interconnected.
– The Light That Shines Through Infinity by Dainin Katagiri

To perform "distance healing" we therefore can use the symbols and mantras to lay bare, even if it is for a split second or a moment, that interconnected state of mind. The state of awareness that our human consciousness is the universe, right now, right this moment. And in that interconnectedness, let the person for whom we are performing "distance healing" take from that state of great bright light whatever they need. No need to label anything, no need to analyze anything at all; let it all go.

Leave your front door and your back door open. Allow your thoughts to come and go. Just don't serve them tea.
– Shunryu Suzuki

This is one of my favorite quotes and teachings – so simple and direct and yet so difficult to do. This is also the essence of Mikao Usui's teachings. Hence whatever thoughts arise, do not cling to them. Let them come and go, just like waves in the sea come and go to the shore and from the shore. Then we are free and we will have a peaceful state of mind.

Chapter 15:

Shinpiden Reiki III

When you help, don't have any notion of being someone who is helping others or any notion of there being an other person who is receiving your help. At that time you can be exactly one with the other person. This is perfect harmony of self and others called oneness.

– The Light That Shines Through Infinity by Dainin Katagiri

Shinpiden means mystery teachings and stands for rediscovering the mystery of ourselves, of the universe. Thus it doesn't point out that we become a teacher, because real teaching comes from our direct experience of emptiness, from our True Self; it is not something we can buy. We can only do this through practice, through integrating Mikao Usui's teachings in our daily life. Mikao Usui taught his students about satori, this has become evident now that we have looked at the previous levels of the system of Reiki. All the teachings point towards this: our right state of mind, that we are infinite light, that we are a divine being, and that we are the precepts.

So the old Gakkai members said that Usui Sensei taught the way to Satori very intensely to those who had achieved a certain level.
– Hiroshi Doi

Of course one can just see the system of Reiki as a hands on/off healing modality and that is perfectly fine. But we cannot deny that Mikao Usui points out again and again our True Self, our non-dual nature, our great bright light. Thus if we really want to be compassionate to ourselves and others, we have to take our practice deeper. We kind of owe it to ourselves and others, as we all live together in this beautiful world.

Fourth Symbol and Mantra

Usui Sensei taught Shinpiden students one on one and he showed them the kanji dai kômyô, which indicated the consciousness of a Shinpiden practitioner.
– Hiroshi Doi, Spain 2015 seminar

This symbol and mantra is a unit just like the third symbol and mantra; the symbol is the kanji of the mantra.

Dai kômyô 大光明
Dai 大 – large, great, big
Kômyô 光明 – hope, glory, bright future
Kô 光 – ray or light
Myô 明 – bright, light, clarity, spell, mantra

Thus dai kômyô 大光明 is our great bright light, our essence, who we truly are, which is emptiness and non-dual in nature. Again we see Mikao Usui pointing this out; thus in each of his levels of teaching, he is pointing to the same aim: laying bare our True Self. Shinpiden Reiki III is not the end; it is where we really start to be serious about our personal spiritual development, the aim of anshin ritsumei – peace of mind, in all we do during our daily life, today.

Your true self is not something separated from others; it is interconnected and constantly working with others. Where? Not in your own small territory, it's working in the huge universe! In Japanese, that working is called Kômyô – light. The functioning energy of the whole world is the light of the self. Because light is working from moment to moment, the whole world constantly manifests itself as the human world. At that time, the whole world

is within the light of the self.
– The Light That Shines Through Infinity by Dainin Katagiri

This wonderful teaching of Zen Master Dainin Katagiri really drives the point home about the light of our True Self: this is interconnectedness and therefore when we work from this state of mind, we are automatically working with others. Automatically, with no need for specific intentions. Just like when we move an arm, the shadow of our arm moves straight away in the same way. There is no gap, no need for setting an intention to move our shadow; it happens simultaneously. This is the same when we lay bare our True Self; compassion is simultaneously for ourselves and others.

Usui Sensei did not give additional healing trainings but I heard that he often taught classes about a Shihan's mental attitude in order to improve one's teaching methods when teaching about healing to the members. Though his one-on-one Shinpi-den lecture did not include healing training, I also heard that Usui Sensei's mentorship greatly enhanced the healing ability of many of the Shinpi-den practitioners, as it strengthened their resonance with the Universe and encouraged the awareness that a human is the small universe derived from the Great Universe.
– Hiroshi Doi

As Hiroshi Doi points out, at this level there is no additional healing training but through the training Mikao Usui taught at this level, the healing ability was greatly enhanced. So what kind of training are we talking about then? Continuing training and practice for the direct experience of our great bright light, emptiness. Because this emptiness is filled with pure energy, which through the direct experience can flow, and emanate freely through our whole body, mind, and speech. This is anshin ritsumei, peace of mind, satori, the direct experience of our human pure mind.

Beyond dualism there is an equality of true human quality. This true quality is the source of actual equality. If we can embrace that, if we can see that equality clearly, then all humans can respect and love each other deeply.
– *Ten Ox Herding Pictures by Zen Master Shodo Harada*

This is what Mikao Usui was teaching, the embodiment of the precepts in all we do. Hence we have to meditate on the symbol and chant the mantra again and again, through which we can reach supreme focus, samatha. So we then can lay bare our great bright light and have insight into our human nature, vipasyana. And through this practice, this process, we lay bare pure love, equality, our true human nature, compassion without change; this is the peace of mind Mikao Usui tried to teach us. Let me recap: it is only through focus, not being distracted by past, present, future that we can lay bare our great bright light. And as we are so often, or maybe always, unfocused, we need to train our mind. We train our mind by using our body and speech, as our mind is very subtle. Hence, we work with the body and speech aspect, as this is a bit easier than working with the mind.

The fourth symbol and mantra is not just used for the reiju. No, not at all: it needs to be embodied in all we do. This means that for today, in every action we do today, and every day, we do it from the mindset of emptiness, non-duality. Even if we live in a dual world, our mind rests in non-duality, and therefore we will experience peace. And it is really from this state of mind that we can perform a reiju. Some Reiki schools do not teach this symbol and mantra, but this is because Mikao Usui taught his students according to their spiritual progress. Hence some of his students were not taught dai kômyô, as they were not ready yet. This makes perfect sense and this is also how many traditional teachers are teaching today. But we can already start at the beginning of our journey with the concept of the great bright light, pointing out our aim. We can do this regardless of how many levels of training we think we might want or might pursue. Through walking the path, practicing all the tools as taught in the three different levels of the system of Reiki, we might hit the target, bullseye right in the middle, right into the heart of non-duality. But even then we have to keep practicing, as our habitual pattern of duality is so ingrained that we have to remind ourselves again and again about our non-dual nature, True Self.

So keep turning the stream of your mind away from your dualistic thoughts and inward to the energy of your life.
– The Light That Shines Through Infinity by Dainin Katagiri

The word meditation really means to familiarize, but now we have to ask ourselves: what are we familiarizing? We are familiarizing ourselves with our inner great bright light, with emptiness, non-duality, so that it will be a continuous awareness in our daily activity, in all we do. Meditation is first of all about acknowledging our innate spaciousness, our innate emptiness, our inner great bright light. This is why we start our practice with freedom, with spaciousness, with the precepts so to speak. With no anger, no worry, with being grateful, with being true to our way and our being, and with compassion to ourselves and others: emptiness.

There are many hidden layers within this symbol and mantra. For example, within the kanji 光 of light we also find fire. By now in our practice, if we practice perfectly, that fire is burning brightly and burns up all our clinging. Then the rain washes away all the residue of what the fire has left, the ash, so that in the end nothing is left. There is no ego clinging, but complete freedom, and emptiness which is compassion and wisdom. But this fire needs to keep burning because we need to keep clearing our clinging. Maybe one day, due to our ongoing practice, we feel this inner bliss through our whole being. And if we cling to this feeling, we just create another attachment. So we have to keep razing all those experiences straight to the ground, clearing and burning, burning and clearing. Only through this can we reveal the ground of our real human nature to ourselves and the world.

All the old masters said the same thing: whatever you are experiencing, however subtle it is, do not cling to it. Be like a bird that flies in the sky; the bird does not leave traces, but is flying in complete emptiness. The more we have the direct experience of emptiness, that great bright light, whatever thought arises will be like writing on water. As soon as you write it, it will disappear, there will be no clinging. And the writing and disappearing happen at the same time! Or in other words, the arising and the disappearing of our thoughts will happen at the same time. This doesn't mean we become zombies, empty-headed and empty-hearted. No, it means that through this emptiness, non-duality, we shine the light of unchangeable compassion, clearly, and wide awake.

Dai kômyô 大光明 in Japan also represents being stable like a mountain. A mountain is stable, it is big, and it is immovable. When you reach the top of a mountain, the view is unlimited, all-encompassing, and our mind is free. And we need to take this state with us in all we do during the day: sleeping, walking, sitting, talking, eating, you name it. This is being stable as a mountain, not moved by anything, fudoshin 不動心 – the mind of fudo. Fudo is a deity in the Japanese esoteric tradition, a personification of being immovable, of emptiness, nothing sticks. And it is from this stage that we have to reenter the dualistic world, to come down from the mountain so to speak, to help other sentient beings to have that same direct experience. This is compassion for yourself and others.

Dualism has to be thrown away as well, or society cannot be truly liberated.
– Ten Ox Herding Pictures by Zen Master Shodo Harada

This is why straight away within Shoden Reiki I, we are pointing ourselves and our students to the realization that we are, right at this moment in time, emptiness, the great bright light. Not tomorrow, or next week, or after one more class, no. Right here today. All of these masters point out the same truth, because it is the universal truth. And therefore, the most important element is to understand the universal truth.

Do not think the moon becomes bright because the clouds move away from it. It has always been bright. Our mind does not become bright because the obstructions are gone. It has always been bright and, even with the clouds in front of it, fully revealed, unmoved.
– Ten Ox Herding Pictures by Zen Master Shodo Harada

Kototama

We discussed the idea behind kototama in a previous chapter, so let's now investigate this specific kototama, the fourth one of the system of Reiki: Dai Kômyô: A I KO YO.

A = Spiritual action – light of life – invisible forces, things we can currently not experience – infinite expansion – all other kototama are born from A – compassion – infinite expansion – unborn – space – universe – also the seed syllable of Dainichi Nyorai, the cosmic Buddha, and therefore it is the origin of all elements – originally non-arising – light of consciousness – gratitude
I = Will of life – center – enlightenment – earth – senses – life force – power – perception
AI = Freedom – love – wisdom – harmony
Ko = Light of spirit – purification of five senses – here and

now – light wave vibration – materialization of Ki
Yo = Light – sometimes like shooting out in one direction like an arrow, like intent. Our intent becomes like the speed of light – purification of the desires created by the five senses – fire/water – the axis between fire and water – the nest (Su) of the fifty sounds

Through the purification of the five senses – smell, touch, sight, hearing, and taste – we start to lay bare the light of our spirit, the great bright light, which is wisdom, compassion, and therefore pure freedom. This light has no beginning and end, just like our mind. Hence this is the mind of enlightenment; it is full of uncontaminated ki. Why the five senses? Because it is through what we see, hear, smell, taste, and touch that we get distracted by the past, present, and future. We interpret, label, distinguish and therefore we move away from experiencing our True Self. But this experience does not come if we chant this mantra once or twice. We first have to prepare the soil, water the plant and give it sunlight, in the right time and the right way; only then can we reap the fruit of laying bare our great bright light, our True Self. So we do this through prolonged chanting of each kototama, step by step. And again, a good teacher can point you to the way, but after the teacher points the way we have to practice ourselves! And if we do not practice the way the teacher instructed, or if we do not practice at all, we will not lay bare the right fruit of the teachings.

Make yourself a light. Rely upon it. Do not depend on anyone else.
– The Light That Shines Through Infinity by Dainin Katagiri

All these Japanese teachings, no matter if it is Zen or Shugendo, point towards this inner light and how important it is in our practice to lay bare this inner light. Because this is the state of mind of peace: real, everlasting peace. And this is why it is of utmost importance to embrace this light, peace, within ourselves. Because it is only through doing this that we can create a peaceful world.

Reiju

So according to Dogen's story, what happens when your clear mirror meets a clear mirror? Both mirrors shatter into pieces, and there is just a great vast openness. That is liberation. You are free. Then next, what should you do? We must not forget re-creation. So come back and pay careful attention to every single aspect of your daily life: getting up in the morning, washing your face, having breakfast, and walking on the street. That is called creating your life. This is very important. Otherwise you cannot take care of your life freely, and you cannot build up a peaceful world.
– The Light That Shines Through Infinity by Dainin Katagiri

What Zen Master Dainin Katagiri points out is a real reiju, when a true teacher who is like a mirror meets a student who is ripe, who also has laid bare their mirror like mind. Then there is a vast openness, full of light and energy, emptiness, liberation. But then we have to go back into our life and share that compassion which we have laid bare. But I jumped the gun here, so let's backtrack a bit and start from the beginning so we can get a better understanding of reiju.

The word reiju really means a spiritual blessing, and this is another part which is so widely misunderstood within Mikao Usui's teachings. Mikao Usui had an enlightened experience on Mount Kurama, so his state of mind was very different from our state of mind as current teachers. This is mainly due to the fact that for most of us, we have not practiced the right way; we have not practiced his teachings in the right order, with the right diligence. And therefore, we have not created a fertile ground for the right fruit to manifest. This in itself is not bad;

we have to start somewhere. But this means that we do not have the right state of mind for a real reiju to take place. The real reiju is performed in that direct experience of emptiness, non-duality, dai kômyô 大光明. This is why Mikao Usui taught this symbol and mantra first in Shinpiden Reiki III, so that we could understand the right state of mind we need to be in for a real reiju to take place. Please let's not fool ourselves and say: "Oh but I am in that state of mind; I can do a real reiju." Please check honestly. Traditionally the teacher would check the student through observation and questions, check their mind, body, speech, to see if they had a direct experience of non-duality. They did this to confirm if the student's experience was real, just imagined or intellectualized. In Zen, for example, if a student claims to have had kensho 見性, seeing one's true nature (the second kanji of kensho is the same as the first kanji of the mantra sei heki), the teacher would check to confirm this.

Anyone who would call himself a member of the Zen family must first of all achieve kensho – realization of the Buddha's way.
– Hakuin on Kensho by Albert Low

And only after the student's kensho was confirmed did they belong to the Zen family, lineage. Now we receive a reiju and we think we belong to the lineage and yet we have no idea what that really means. True lineage within Mikao Usui's teachings is reached through the direct confirmed experience of seeing our own great bright light, dai kômyô 大光明; then we can truly say that we are practicing in the lineage of Mikao Usui in the way that his teachings point out. And at that stage we also see no need to change Mikao Usui's teachings.

Thus a real reiju has the potential to trigger a direct experience of our great bright light, emptiness, within ourselves. But if the teacher is not in that state of mind then it would already be, almost, impossible for a student to have this direct experience.

If, however, the teacher is in that state of mind, then there is a possibility. But that all depends on the student.

The three defects of the student. One is like an upside-down vase that nothing can enter; another is a like a vase with a hole in it in which nothing that is poured in remains inside, and the third is like a dirty vase, whatever you put into it is mixed with poisons and emotions.

– Namkhai Norbu

Thus a real reiju from a real teacher, who is in that state of mind of emptiness, will help the student, who is like an empty vase, to see what they already are from beginningless time: emptiness, non-duality. Due to our habitual patterns, that experience will only last for a moment before we come back to what we think of as "reality". But it will leave a trace, a taste so to speak, like if we stick our tongue in a good glass of wine but then don't drink it. Now the student can recall this taste again and again and that is what they use to meditate upon: this is true meditation, familiarizing ourselves with emptiness because we have tasted it. The aim of the path is non-duality, emptiness, our great bright light, and a student who has this direct experience during reiju can take the aim as the path. They practice the aim, they practice with non-duality, with no-form, but that can only happen if they have that direct experience. This is the highest form of reiju. So please let us not fool ourselves and think we have received this or that we are giving this kind of reiju. Please be careful, else we will only prolong our path. We may get there; we may not. But we must be honest with ourselves in our practice, and we must practice to move honestly on our path.

However, the one who says he is enlightened – calling himself enlightened, that is unfortunate. That person is most likely deluded. He is making a great mistake.

– Discovering the True Self by Kōdō Sawaki

As we are not always an empty vase, a ripe student, we might not have that direct experience, and therefore we have meditation practices like chanting, breathing methods, symbols to focus on. And through practicing these we become an empty vase, the right vase, so that when a real teacher performs a reiju again on us we might have that direct experience of emptiness. Now our whole practice will change, our whole perception will change. Now we practice the inner teachings of Mikao Usui, the essence.

Someone then asked, "What does realization all at once mean?" Hakuin answered that when the discriminating mind is suddenly shattered and the awakened essence immediately appears, the universe is filled with its boundless light. This is called the way of knowing of the Great Perfect Mirror, the pure body of reality.
– Hakuin on Kensho by Albert Low

This is why emptiness is often compared to a mirror. The mirror reflects everything and yet does not get caught up in what it reflects, with no intellectual interpretation, no clinging, no labelling; it just reflects what is. Things come and go and the mirror does not lament. This is the mirror mind of the great bright light, dai kômyô 大光明, my original nature is right mind, our infinite light, our natural disposition, being a divine being, direct spirit, and of the embodiment of the precepts. But even at this stage you have to keep practicing, because the mirror can get dusty again, and we can always go deeper. Thus even if we can meditate directly on emptiness, we also need mantras, symbols, etc. due to our habitual dual patterns. And that is why we work with form and no-form in our practice.

Let's explore reiju a bit more. First we establish that reiju is the Japanese word for the initiation or attunement we perform within the Reiki system. In Japan, there is just one word for these rituals; initiation and attunement are the English translations we have given to the word reiju. There are different styles of reiju in Japan. Some are very simple (without symbols or mantras), and some are very elaborate (with symbols and mantras). Mikao Usui based the ritual of reiju on existing Japanese esoteric practices, which he was practicing himself at the time. The common touch-points are the crown, forehead/ eyes, throat, heart, the shoulders/side of the head, and hands. In the Japanese esoteric tradition, these points are used to attain identification with a specific deity. To paraphrase a Japanese esoteric ritual manual, by using the hand to touch the self [and others] on these key points of the eyes, heart, throat, and so on, the body is considered to become transformed into (and divinely empowered by) the invoked deity. Of course, we first have to learn how to empower ourselves before we can truly empower others. This is why dai kômyô is all about self-empowerment, the direct experience of emptiness. Within the system of Reiki, the symbol/mantra dai kômyô points to this deity, Dainichi Nyorai. Dainichi Nyorai is the personification of the cosmos. Thus, in other words, we can say that through the focus on these key points during the ritual of reiju, we attain identification with the cosmos. Not only does dai kômyô point to this – the other symbols and mantras used within the system of Reiki do also. This doesn't mean we have to become Buddhists or believe in those deities, all it means is that we realize that we are the cosmos. Someone might say that they now feel a deep union with God or that they are the Tao; these are just different words for the same thing.

The meditation upon selflessness, and specifically the meditation upon the lack of true existence of the personal self, is done by replacing your solid sense of your own existence with something else. In the case of the Medicine Buddha practice, this consists of imagining yourself to be the Medicine Buddha, conceiving of yourself as the Medicine Buddha. By replacing the thought of yourself as your ordinary self with the thought of yourself as the Medicine Buddha, you gradually counteract and remove the fixation on your personal self.

– Medicine Buddha Teachings by Khenchen Thrangu Rinpoche

This identification with a deity is a widespread practice within the Japanese esoteric traditions and is often called nyuga ga 'nya – deity entering self, self entering deity. In Japanese esoteric ritual manuals, it is explained that "having gained ritualized union with the deity, the practitioner attains the empowerment of kaji (kaji: union, Buddha's power transferred to sentient beings) and is now able to manipulate the powers of the deity and fulfil the objectives of the ritual." So what are these "powers" used for? And what are these powers? These powers are wisdom and compassion and are used for healing and empowerment, just like we do within the system of Reiki. But of course, this unification is easier said than done. This is why we need to practice and receive reiju repeatedly until we attain full identification with the cosmos. And this might take the rest of our lives. And it is thus only at the stage of full unification with the cosmos that we can perform true reijus!

Strict teachings and rules of Master Usui: One of the most strict rules which he taught us is that your spirit as a small universe has to be always united with the spiritual power of the whole universe as one.

– Reiki Ryôhô no Shiori which is handed out by the Usui Reiki Ryôhô Gakkai

When we first enter the teaching in Shoden Reiki I we receive four reijus, depending on the structure of the teachings. Thus in a way if we are ripe, an empty vase, and the teacher is in the right mind state of emptiness themselves, then there is a possibility that right at the beginning of our journey we can have a direct taste, experience, of emptiness. But even if we have that we still have to practice, because it is only a glimpse.

Awakening is not an experience; it is a change in the way we experience. Many people confuse an experience of unity and completeness with awakening. This is why we must have an awakening authenticated by a teacher. Any experience – even the most intense, meaningful, and transformative – is not awakening.
– Hakuin on Kensho by Albert Low

Now when we have looked at the deeper aspects of reiju we also come to the conclusion that when we are performing a reiju, we are not giving anything to anybody at all. We are not opening up a person's energy field and we are not opening or activating a chakra, or energy center. We are also not giving them Reiki, their True Self, which is impossible because how can we give a person their True Self?! First of all why not? Because dai kômyô stands for non-duality; thus in the state of reiju there is no "I" and therefore also no "you". This means there is nothing to give or do. We have to understand this very clearly and carefully if we want to practice from Mikao Usui's viewpoint, which he so elegantly pointed out within his teachings.

Light is the original nature of your life. Everyone has that light.
– The Light That Shines Through Infinity by Dainin Katagiri

How can I give you light if you are already light? I can only help you to rediscover this and that is what hands on/off healing and reiju are all about. Practices to help others to rediscover their own inner great bright light, the light which they already have. Thus there is nothing to give.

Teaching

Zen Master Hakuin said: "The only worry is that real teachers of Zen are extremely few and hard to find." Sorry to say this, but not really sorry; we can say the same for Reiki teachers. Real teaching comes from our direct experience of our True Self, not from reading a book and/or attending a lecture. Doing these and repeating what you have read and learned to others without putting in the time and the practice, and working to understand what it all means, that is just being a parrot. Some people may just want to do a Reiki course to be able to teach or open up a center to do hands on/off healing on others, but that is the wrong motivation. Our motivation needs to be first of all that we want to lay bare our great bright light. If we just do it to make money, then it is better that we stop right now. Because it is not going to happen, and if it happens it is like the blind leading the blind.

Teaching the system of Reiki is also not teaching from something we have created, it needs to come from the source, the natural. Many teachers will say, I created this and that kind of teachings and/or lineage, but that is not the way of Reiki as it was intended to be taught. That is created by the confused mind. To really teach, we have to teach from the un-created, from our natural source. What is this natural source? It is emptiness, non-duality, pure compassion. Why do we have to teach from this natural source? Because when we teach that way we are free of attachments, free of strings. And therefore we do not, as teachers, get tied up in our own attachment and we are not tying others with the strings of attachments. The most important teaching we can offer is the ultimate truth; this truth is uncreated, free of confused human dualistic ideas. If we teach duality then we put the student on the path of duality, which means they will stay confused, get easily angry and worried, and therefore the teachings will take them deeper into suffering. The teachings need to be focused, straight from the beginning on non-duality, the ultimate truth, so that the students can have peace of mind in their daily life. So in Shoden Reiki I, we already point towards non-duality, the great bright light; that is the base of the teachings. We kind of put the students' noses towards the aim, else they will walk completely in the wrong direction.

Usui Sensei had no standard curriculum, and the length of time of the training depended on the spiritual progress of each student.
– Hiroshi Doi

Over time we have put the teachings in narrow boxes, and therefore we get a narrow understanding. Better to teach the students according to their own personal progress, each student is unique in that way, we cannot teach the system of Reiki cookie cutter style.

Teach individuals one by one. Rather than educating people generally within a system, we need to address each individually, since each is unique.
– Discovering the True Self by Kōdō Sawaki

Thus, how do we teach others? By first gaining a direct experience, again, and again, of all the methods and practices, so that we know them by heart and also know all the pitfalls of the practice. That we have an understanding of the teachings as a whole, what their aim is, how to explain this aim, how to guide a student towards this aim, teaching from the essence. Then when students come with questions we can focus on the essence and the answers will manifest themselves. This is why we can place the filter of the precepts and non-duality over each question, as they are the essence of the system of Reiki. When we teach, there are people listening; thus our speech needs to be clear. Our speech will be clear if we have harmonized it with our mind and body. If our mind is all over the place, our speech will be all over the place and the student will not have a clear understanding of what we are saying. As teachers we also have to come to the students' level, as each student is unique. And so each teaching, if we teach individuals, is unique. In a class, we may explain things in different ways, depending on the students' level or understanding: we meet them where they are.

If we treat things as they should be without being upset by our surroundings and without letting our minds be dispersed by them under any circumstances, we may be called masters wherever we may be.
– Introduction to Zen Training: A Physical Approach to Meditation and Mind-Body Training by Omori Sogen

This is why I find it is much better to call ourselves teachers rather than masters. If we haven't cut our own clinging yet, how can we be masters? Then we are just pretending to ourselves and others; we have bought a certificate but in our mind, body, speech we are not masters at all. I see some teachers becoming upset by their students, their students' questions, or their students' behavior. But if we as teachers get upset, that really shows that we are not masters at all as we haven't even mastered what we are teaching! When we have a problem with another, we blame that person but if we understand that everything is interconnected, hon sha ze sho nen, I am Right Mind, then we will realize that we ourselves, as teachers, are also part of that problem.

Often teachers want to teach in a specific style but when we get stuck to that style we are not natural anymore. The teachings are not coming from emptiness, which means open-minded and flexible. Else we teach like an ice cube, instead of like free flowing water which can fit in any kind of shape. Again this is why we have to teach from the foundation, and in Mikao Usui's teaching that is non-duality, emptiness, as he pointed out again and again within his teachings and practices.

What you invent cannot really be called a teaching. Today, in modern society, we have so many methods belonging to the New Age style. Many people say that this is very good because they can produce certain benefits. Maybe, relatively speaking, there may be some benefit, but it is only a relative type of benefit.
– Namkhai Norbu

Thus to really teach, we have to do our best and sit on our butt to have the direct experience of what we are trying to teach and to point out to our students. And this is the embodiment of the precepts.

It is generally said that it takes ten years to master one art. Therefore, it is necessary to be trained continually for a considerable number of years in order to master any skill, however trivial it may seem.
– *Introduction to Zen Training: A Physical Approach to Meditation and Mind-Body Training by Omori Sogen*

In November of 2019, I was part of an international group of Reiki practitioners and teachers exploring Japan and Mikao Usui's teachings. During this journey we were fortunate to experience different traditional Japanese ceremonies, from tea ceremony to the esoteric ritual of Goma, from Mikkyo chanting rituals to kaji – blessings, and from Shinto blessing to Shinto chanting. One important thing which stood out for me is that these traditional teachers practiced in such a different way than many modern teachers do. We can learn a lot from observing these rituals.

The first point is that they practiced these rituals with such focus, not being distracted by past, present, and future. There was no gap between their practice and their state of mind.

Without such a gap, their rituals cut straight to the core, the core of their being. And as we all are interconnected, with no real gap between these traditional teachers and us, their practice therefore creates a possibility of also cutting straight to our being. Thus every ritual they performed had the potential of being an empowerment, a blessing. Why the potential and not the result? Because the person watching the ritual also needs as much as possible to be in a state of mind of not being distracted by past, present, and future. As the Zen saying goes: you can't pour anything into a full cup.

There is such a difference when we see many modern rituals being performed; often there is a big gap between the ritual and the mind – they are not one. Between the ritual and the focused mind is a mind that for us is distracted by past, present, and future. Like the full cup, our minds are too busy and distracted to be fully open.

The second point with these traditional teachers was that after their ritual was performed, they all stayed in emptiness. What does that mean, staying in emptiness? Zen master Dainin Katagiri describes staying in emptiness this way: that there is no "stickiness" or "stink" left after what you have practiced. What this stickiness or stink is, is all about the ego: look what I just did! I just performed this great ritual, I can do this and you can't, I saw this or that, I am special, let me tell you what I saw or felt... I, I, I. You know what this kind of stickiness is; it is our ego boost, trying to show off, trying to be special. But these teachers just performed these rituals and boom... finished. No stickiness or stink left. By staying in emptiness, emptiness which had deepened during the ritual, they had no stickiness or stink left, and thus after the performed ritual they stay free.

This freedom is spiritual freedom which helps them to go even deeper into their practice. But when we have a stickiness left we can't move to the deeper layers, as we are stuck in our ego boosting. That trip was therefore one great big lesson for me:

to practice more, so that there will be no gap between my mind and body when I live my life. It was a lesson to practice more so that there will be no stickiness or stink left after whatever I do, whether it is a hands on/off healing session, teaching a class or at a retreat, performing a ritual or just living my day-to-day life. It was a lesson to become a better teacher for, as long as we are here, we always can improve. So please do not think that because you have bought a piece of paper that states you are a Reiki Master, now you do not have to practice anymore. That is delusion, and it robs you of the many benefits your practice can bring, for you and for others.

This Taoist verse points out very clearly how we need to teach:

Therefore the Master acts without doing anything
and teaches without saying anything.
Things arise and she lets them come;
things disappear and she lets them go.
She has but doesn't possess,
acts but doesn't expect.
When her work is done, she forgets it.
That is why it lasts forever.
– Tao Te Ching: a new English version, by Stephen Mitchell

This verse is all about emptiness: no clinging, no strings attached. And it is from that state of mind, body, and speech that we need to teach. Of course the master does something, the master acts, but because the act comes out of emptiness it feels like they are not doing anything. It is natural and not artificial, not created. Of course the teacher says something, but because they speak from emptiness nothing gets stuck. Thus it feels like they are not saying anything, like drawing words upon water. Things come and things go, no clinging to whatever happens: freedom. The real master has it but there is no proclamation like, look at me, look what I have got, showing off, standing on a pedestal. There are no expectations, thus they are free, utterly free. When the work is done, any activity in their daily life, it is forgotten because there is not clinging. And that is why it lasts forever.

This verse really describes the fourth precept: be true to our way and our being. This is how our life needs to be, and how we can see if we are still in a dualistic state of mind. And therefore this points to the state of mind of a true master. Now we can check for ourselves: are we in that state of mind? Do we let things come and go? Do we expect things from our students? Can we let things go when they say our teachings suck or when they do not agree with something we explain? After we have been teaching, do we need to keep talking about it, do we keep thinking about the class or can we let it go? This is what we have to check very honestly within ourselves. Maybe we say we can do all this, but that might be on a good day, when we are praised as a teacher. Because if that is what we see as a good day, then we are clinging again to being praised. So check carefully, honestly.

In ultimate emptiness there are no ideas, no concepts, not even of emptiness.
– The Light That Shines Through Infinity by Dainin Katagiri

Communication

As teacher we have to communicate clearly, so let's look at how we can make this happen. We communicate in so many ways, on so many levels: physical, verbal, nonverbal, speaking from the gut or through the written word... you can probably think of more. But within all these different levels of communication is one very important element: how we communicate with ourselves. Communication with others is in fact based on how we communicate with ourselves. For very clear communication, first we need to be very clear within our own mind. If our own mind is all over the place, our communication with others also will be all over the place. If I want to communicate my thoughts or feelings to others in a loving way, if I want to communicate with others in a loving way, I first have to love myself. How can I love others if I do not love myself? Or as I always say, how can I give you tea if I do not have tea?

Of course we all want to be in and to communicate from a place of love. But we might communicate in an angry way or react angrily to what someone says or does because we haven't made peace within ourselves yet. When we are not communicating within ourselves in a peaceful way, that is reflected in our communication not only with others (having a dialogue) but also to others (telling them something). Peaceful internal communication is important for either situation. But what does communicating within ourselves in a peaceful way look like?

One of the first elements of this is to love our own physical being, as that is the vehicle for our mind. If we are constantly saying things like – whether in words or our own thoughts – "I do not like this aspect of my physicality, I am not happy with the way my body is, I do not like my grey hair, my scar, my long hands," then we are constantly communicating ideas to ourselves in a way that is not healthy for our mind or body. This kind of communication within ourselves therefore will be reflected in how and what we communicate to others. Thus, we need to learn how to accept our whole physical being no matter what, and to communicate this acceptance to our own physicality in a loving and caring way. This is being grateful for our physical body, the vehicle for our mind and energy. Just as our physical being is the vehicle for our mind, our mind often is the driver of our feelings. And when we love our own physical body deeply, we can then start to work on our feelings.

Often we do not express our own feelings in an open and

kind way to ourselves, let alone to others. We might hide our emotions due to feeling ashamed of what we feel. For example, you watch a movie and feel like crying but you feel ashamed to do this. Maybe you learned as a child that crying was a sign of weakness or was "bad", or that the feeling of wanting to cry was something to push down or to close off in a corner of your mind. Maybe there are other things that you close off in your mind, that you close off from your communications.

The more we open our mind, the more free it will become and the more we will start to communicate with our own feelings in a more open and loving way, with compassion and acceptance from that state of emptiness. The more we accept our own feelings and communicate clearly with them, the more we can communicate more clearly, freely, and compassionately with others.

But even if our mind is open as wide as can be, we need to look after our body, feelings and emotions as well, as all are connected and all can affect our communication. For example, when we feel tired within ourselves, we might get angry more quickly than if we feel well rested. Or when we feel emotionally unstable, we might more easily get angry or worried.

Therefore, clear communication with ourselves and others comes from being stable within our own physical being, which means we are centered and grounded in our own physicality. Then through this centeredness we start to communicate more clearly with our own personal feelings and emotions. And this in turn will help us to communicate with and to others in a very clear, kind, open-minded way. Hence the first step to learn how to communicate in a loving and clear way to others is to learn how to communicate in a loving and clear way to ourselves.

In order to be effective in benefiting other beings, we need to accomplish an excellent samadhi or meditative absorption. In order to have this stable and profound practice, we need to be physically and mentally healthy or comfortable, so we will be free of obstacles to diligence in practice and free of obstacles to the cultivation of meditative absorption.

– The Practice of Tranquillity and Insight by Khenchen Thrangu Rinpoche

Khenchen Thrangu puts it very elegantly, that to really benefit other beings we have to be in that state of emptiness: no attachment, no clinging, free of confused dualistic ideas. We need to be physically and mentally healthy and comfortable within our own body/mind, else we just bring our own issues to the teachings. We have to practice diligently, just like Mikao Usui said, to be able to stay in that state of mind when we are teaching. This is not done through just ticking a box, but through constant daily meditation practice. Therefore a good teacher teaches from their mind, body, and speech, sanmitsu.

Chapter 16:

History

This is not really a history book but rather a practical book, on how to practice. We can read about the history of Mikao Usui in many different books. Of course the history is important but also a slippery slope as we can view history from many angles, especially because there is not much known about the man himself. However, the real history of Mikao Usui can be found in the practices: the mantras, the words he used, the teachings he showed his students. This for me is so much more important because they point to why we practice and how we need to practice. As we have seen already, Mikao Usui's teachings are really based on Japanese spiritual practices like Zen, Shugendo, Tendai, and Shinto. Let's now look at kaji, an ancient Japanese esoteric practice which bears lots of similarities with Mikao Usui's teachings. And let's look at the kanji of Reiki and its history, because when we do this we can start to see clearly why Mikao Usui used this kanji in his teachings. But remember, it is only through practice that we can have a direct experience of what Mikao Usui was pointing out to us: our True Self, emptiness, our great bright light, the embodiment of the precepts. This does not happen through intellectualizing or debating the history. In this chapter we look at the heritage of Mikao Usui's teachings and also the heritage of the word Reiki. Examining these can help us get a clearer idea on why and how to practice. And then, as we know is so important, we practice!

Kaji

Kaji is a practice within Japanese esoteric traditions which is about enlightenment, healing, initiation, blessing, empowerment, and often is performed for a person who is not physically present. Within the system of Reiki we see the same elements: enlightenment, healing, initiation, blessing, empowerment. We also see something which in the modern system of Reiki is called "distance" healing and is performed for a person who is not physically present. Did Mikao Usui base his teachings on this ancient Japanese practice of kaji?

Kaji for Self

One beautiful translation of kaji 加持 is given by Kukai: "Ka is the sun of the Buddha reflected in the water of the mind of all beings. And ji means the water of the practitioner's mind experiencing the sun of the Buddha." Another wonderful translation of kaji is by Ryuko Oda: "Kaji (Sk: adhisthana) is the transference of the Buddha's power or grace which inspires a sacred peace of mind and a strengthening of the life force." In other words, kaji is about realizing that you and Buddha are one and the same, which is called nyū ga gan yū – 入我我入.

In kaji, the main Buddha with whom you realize union is Dainichi Nyorai – the cosmic Buddha, often also translated as "The Great Illuminating One" or "Life Force That Illuminates the Universe". Or as Ryuko Oda points out, "Dainichi Nyorai personifies the essential nature of the universe and also symbolizes the wisdom and compassion which allows us to realize the true world of our mind."

Within Shinpiden Reiki Level III we learn the mantra and symbol dai kômyô (lit: Great Bright Light) which is traditionally linked to Dainichi Nyorai. Thus Mikao Usui was pointing out that through practicing the meditations taught within the system of Reiki, we can realize this unification with dai kômyô – the Great Bright Light – which in essence is nothing different from Dainichi Nyorai, the essential nature of the universe which is wisdom and compassion. Thus Mikao Usui pointed out the same as what we find within the kaji teachings.

However, realizing this state of union is not so easy to do.

We really can only do it through long and dedicated practice. This is why traditionally the system of Reiki was a lifelong meditation practice.

... kaji is quite often a synonym for yuga, or union. This refers to the understanding that Buddha and sentient life are not separate, but are connected and interfused... Such awakening is initially temporary, but through focused and sustained practice the priest can sustain this state, which is essential for the maturing of practice. When honzon kaji can be sustained beyond the ritual, the practitioner truly becomes one with the honzon [main object of veneration]. At this point the practitioner is in the samadhi (Sanskrit: contemplation) of the three secrets (san mitsu) and has entered the state of funi (not two).
– What is Kaji by Shingon Priest Eijun Eidson

Here Eijun Eidson is pointing out sanmitsu which we have seen also is pointed out within Mikao Usui's teachings. He also is pointing out that meditative state of mind of emptiness, as Mikao Usui also often did, pointing out that we have to maintain this in all we do, today, beyond the ritual. Thus we can say in a way that when we fully rediscover that we are Reiki, Buddha, our True Self, Kami, the essential nature of the universe, then we experience real kaji, the real blessing.

This power [Kaji] is held by those who realize a state of enlightenment realized by Shakyamuni Buddha, as well as by those who strive in their life-style to understand and know the truth he discovered.
– Kaji: Empowerment and Healing in Esoteric Buddhism by Ryuko Oda

Mikao Usui also said, "We humans hold the Great Reiki that fills the Great Universe. The higher we raise the vibration of our own being, the stronger the Reiki we have inside will be." Thus we can gradually start to see that the practice of kaji is very similar to Mikao Usui's deeper teachings.

Kaji for Others

When the practitioner works towards and realizes this union, they also could start to perform kaji for others.

In addition to the changes that kaji confers on the practitioner, it also has healing qualities. In both ancient and modern times, kaji healing has been performed to assist a person who is ill.
— What is Kaji by Shingon Priest Eijun Eidson

Here we can see the same in what Mikao Usui was teaching us. When we remember our great bright light, dai kômyô, it will change us, and that change has healing qualities. And because we are compassionate to others, we can assist a person who is ill.

There are many rituals a priest or priestess can perform for kaji when a person asks for healing. Some are very elaborate and last hours, while in others the priest or priestess simply touches the body at specific places. These rituals depend on the state of mind of the performer and on the state of mind of the person who is seeking healing. Sometimes there is no ritual at all; the priest or priestess sits opposite the person seeking healing and allows it to take place, just as it is said that Mikao Usui did when he performed Reiju. I have personally "received" kaji from different priests while in Japan and in Japanese temples outside of Japan. Some took a long time with lots of chanting and even a fire ritual, while others were a simple ritual in which the priest touched me at different points. What is interesting to note is that when the priests touched me during these elaborate or simple rituals, they touched the same places as we do in reiju! Hence we can see many overlapping elements within kaji and the system of Reiki.

As kaji healing is all about union with the universe, the priest or priestess realizes that there is no receiver, giver, and gift during the ritual. This is exactly the same as what Mikao Usui pointed out within his own teachings. Within Okuden Reiki II the mantra and symbol Hon Sha Ze Sho Nen 本者 points towards this non-dual thought, as does dai kômyô within his Shinpiden Reiki III teachings.

One other very important element is pointed out by Ryuko Oda: "Spiritual healing, Kaji in Esoteric Buddhism, is not a medical practice. Its principal purpose is to provide a sacred peace of mind."

This of course is the same within the system of Reiki, and Mikao Usui pointed this out with the precepts: peace of mind. Healing is all about a state of mind in which there is no anger, no worry; it is about being grateful, true to our way and our being and being compassionate, thus creating a sacred peace of mind. Because it is through this sacred peace of mind that healing starts to take place. All these teachers were pointing out the same: that the mind is the crux of the practice and that we use the body and speech/breath/energy to support this practice to create Right Mind.

Due to this deep understanding of what Mikao Usui called Hon Sha Ze Sho Nen – my original nature is a non-dual thought – the priest or priestess also performs kaji for people who are not physically present. But they do not call it "distance" healing, as they know that in that state of mind of union with the universe that there is no distance at all. As we can now slowly start to see, there are many similarities between kaji and Mikao Usui's teachings. However, the way we practice the system of Reiki from a modern perspective does not resemble much of kaji, as often it is all externalized and not internalized. Therefore we need to check what our aim is and how we can stimulate real, deep healing within ourselves and others, cutting straight to the root, laying bare our empty state of mind, our True Self. There are many more elements which suggest that Mikao Usui based his teachings on kaji, but they need to be taught in person by a teacher well-versed in these practices.

So the more we start to see what Mikao Usui practiced himself, the more we start to get a clearer idea of what his own teachings were based on. Understanding is important but by itself is not enough. As practitioners and students of the system of Reiki, we need to practice daily the meditation practices Mikao Usui put into his teachings. We need to practice daily so that we can have a direct experience of this union, this great bright light – dai kômyô – the embodiment of the precepts. We need to practice daily so that we, ultimately, can have a peaceful mind.

Reiki in Ancient China

Prior to when kanji was used within Japan it existed already in China. So how was the kanji and concept of Reiki 靈氣 used in ancient China and how does it relate to the teachings of Mikao Usui?

As we know, this Dao or Dao-Qi 道氣 tends to radiate itself and permeate the whole universe with itself as Jing-Qi 精氣 or Ling-Qi 靈氣.
– Re-figuring St. Thomas's Concept of Ipsum Esse Subsistens in terms of the Concept of Qi in the Guanzi's Four Daoist Chapters
– John Cheng

靈氣 means Ling Chi, Ling Ch'i or Ling Qi in Chinese. It is a Taoist concept and just like the system of Reiki, is a practice to lay bare our inner great bright light, the Tao.

Ling Chi is the subtlest and most highly refined of all the energies in the human system and the product of the most advanced

stages of practice, whereby the ordinary energies of the body are transformed into pure spiritual vitality.
– Harnessing the Power of the Universe: A Complete Guide to the Principles and Practice of Chi-Gung by Daniel Reid

Within the quote by Daniel Reid, we can see that Ling Chi 靈氣 is the "most highly and refined of all energies in the human system." Here he is pointing out that it is first of all inside of us, just as Mikao Usui pointed out that Reiki is first of all inside of us. Both noted that we have to practice to transform our ordinary energies into pure spiritual vitality, in Mikao Usui's case, Reiki 靈氣. The ordinary energies of anger and worry are transmuted into the energy of pure compassion through chanting the precepts, meditation practices, hands on/off healing, internalizing the symbols and mantras – all of our practices within the system of Reiki.

That being said, let us look at what Ling is. Ling is considered an expression of the more evolved aspects of spirit when it functions in the realm of manifestation. It is said that Ling Shen (靈神) – "magical spirit manifest through human mind" – produces Ling Qi (靈氣), the "expressed energy of the Ling". This Qi then results in the production of Siddhi which may manifest within a practitioner.
– A Comprehensive Guide to Daoist Nei Gong by Damo Mitchell

Damo Mitchell points out that Ling Qi 靈氣 is a product – expression of Ling Shen, magical spirit manifested through the human mind. Of course when our mind lets go of anger and worry, we can manifest Ling Qi 靈氣. Again, Mikao Usui pointed this out too: we can see it clearly within the precepts, which are all about the mind. But we also can see that the mind is really important for that expression of Reiki in the mantras. (Remember, one translation of Hon Sha Ze Sho Nen 本者是正念 is my original nature is right mind.)

Damo Mitchell goes further to say that this Qi results in the production of siddhi; siddhi is the accomplishment of perfect realization of our spiritual practice. Thus 靈氣 helps us to accomplish realization. It supports us through the transformation in our body and mind so that we can lay bare our True Self, our great bright light.

> ... the Transmutation of Vapor into Spiritual Energy, or ling-ch'i [靈氣]. The mundane breath is transformed into Spiritual Energy. Ling-ch'i [靈氣] is formless and can be channeled to the internal organs and all parts of the body. When the body is filled with this energy, the state is known as the Five Vapors Gathering at the Origin.
> – Cultivating Stillness: A Taoist Manual for Transforming Body and Mind – translated with an introduction by Eva Wong (Cultivating Stillness was written 220-589 CE)

The ancient manual of *Cultivating Stillness* also points out that we are transforming our energy into ling-ch'i 靈氣 and that we can channel this to the internal organs and all parts of our body. Through this transformation, our whole body will be filled with ling-ch'i 靈氣. Mikao Usui taught us the meditation practice of hatsurei-ho, which literally translates as a "method to emit our hidden inconceivable spiritual ability". Thus hatsurei-ho, this specific meditation practice, parallels what *Cultivating Stillness* described thousands of years ago.

> The three treasures are also known as the three flowers, the three jewels, or the three herbs. They are ching (generative energy), ch'i (vital energy or vapor) and shen (spiritual energy, or ling-ch'i [靈氣]). These three energies were originally uncontaminated when we were in our mother's womb. In their pure form they are "original generative energy," "original vapor," and "original

spirit." When we breathe earthly air, engage in sexual activity, think and become attached to things in the world, ch'i, ching, and shen become impure, thus losing their Earlier Heaven quality. The aim of the internal alchemical process is to gather and recover these three energies, refine them, and transform them to the original state. The process of refinement is labeled the gathering of the three flowers (or herbs) in the cauldron, the cauldron being the crucible where the refinement takes place. The stove is the generator and the cauldron is the crucible where the refinement of the three energies takes place. In the purification of the three treasures, the lower tan-t'ien is the stove.

– Cultivating Stillness: A Taoist Manual for Transforming Body and Mind – translated with an introduction by Eva Wong (Cultivating Stillness was written 220-589 CE)

Again we see that to really lay bare our ling-ch'i 靈氣 – our Reiki 靈氣 – we need to practice. We can't just think, talk, or write about it. We need to sit on our butt and meditate, so that the transformation can take place, remembering what we have lost, recovering what we have lost. What have we lost? Our True Self, our great bright light which emanates 靈氣. Or in Usui's words, we have lost how to be compassionate because we have focused on our anger and worry. And the first point of call, as *Cultivating Stillness* and Mikao Usui both point out, is the hara – tan-t'ien – just below our navel. Mikao Usui placed specific meditation practices in his system like jōshin kokyū hō and seishin toitsu in which we focus our mind and breath/energy on the hara – tan-t'ien.

This concept of getting distracted by our anger and worry and practicing to regain our spiritual energy/essence, ling ch'i – Reiki 靈氣, is clearly visible in the ancient text of Nei-Ye 內業 which was written around 350-300 BCE. Nei-Ye stands for Inner Cultivation and was written in verses. One verse clearly describes the concept of anger and worry and 靈氣.

The original Chinese text of this verse is below:

凡人之生也, 必以其歡, 憂則失紀, 怒則失端, 憂悲喜怒, 道乃無處, 愛慾靜之, 遇亂正之 勿引勿推, 福將自歸 彼道自來, 可藉與謀 靜則得之, 躁則失之, 靈氣在心, 一來一逝 其細無內, 其大無外, 所以失之, 以躁為害, 心能執靜, 道將自定 得道之人, 理丞而屯泄, 匈中無敗 節欲之道, 萬物不害

Here is the translation as found in *Anthology of Daoist Texts: Selections of Key Scriptures, Commentaries, and Other Historical Documents*:

The lives of all people. Must have happiness. When anxious, they lose their reason; When angry, they lose their direction. (If people are hindered by) anxiety, grief, euphoria, and anger, Dao is then without any (empty) place to abide. Attachment and lust: quiet them; Encountering confusion, correct it. Do not pull, do not push. Then good fortune will approach and naturally return. This Dao of (allowing good fortune to) approach spontaneously. Can be relied on by following this strategy: If tranquil, you will attain it; If agitated, you will lose it; The magical energy-breath (ling qi) within the heart-mind: For a moment it draws near, and the next it disperses. So thin, there is nothing inside of it; So wide, there is nothing outside of it. The reason you lose it. Is that agitation obstructs it. If the heart-mind can remain quiet, Dao will approach and (ling qi will) naturally affix itself. People who attain Dao. Are aided by its principles, which fill and flow through them. Within the breast, they are not defeated (by pleasure, anger, sadness, or worry). Applying the dao of restraining the desires (of the five senses), The myriad things do not harm them.

(See two more translations from different sources of this text further on.)

For me, I can clearly see Mikao Usui's teachings within this verse. And again we can see that ling qi 靈氣 is within the mind, just like Mikao Usui pointed out, and that the reason we are not aware of this ling qi is that we are distracted by anger and worry. Hence we need to practice the meditation practices which Mikao Usui put in his teachings so that we can calm our mind, with no agitation. We need to practice so that we can reach a state of emptiness, pure tranquility, Right Mind, a state of not being distracted by the five senses.

By looking at these ancient Chinese practices and how the Taoists saw the concept of ling qi 靈氣 we can see how this interlaces with Mikao Usui's teachings. We should of course not forget that Taoism also was integrated within Japanese spiritual practices, such as Onmyōdō and Shugendō.

To sum it all up, we have to transmute our worry and anger, as pointed out within the Reiki precepts. We have to transmute our worry and anger into pure compassion, and the essence of this compassion is in reality Reiki 靈氣. But of course that is easier said than done, and again that is why Mikao Usui put meditation practices within his system to help us still our confused mind. This in turn will enable us to shine the light of our True Self – Reiki 靈氣 – forward in all we do. Within the full text of the Reiki precepts Mikao Usui also wrote: *shinshin kaizen* 心身改善 – improve your mind/body. Thus he was pointing out the improvement of our mind and body through the transformation of our mundane energy into Reiki 靈氣 in our mind and body. Some of this may look simple but it is not that easy, as there are many hidden layers within these texts and Mikao Usui's teachings. A qualified teacher who has walked/is walking this path themselves can help guide you through these inner teachings, guide you through this process of transformation.

Gradually, the golden xin 金心 *of a sage becomes, then, an immense qi reservoir* 氣淵 *of Jing-Qi* 精氣 *or Ling-Qi* 靈氣*.*
– Re-figuring St. Thomas's Concept of Ipsum Esse Subsistens in

*terms of the Concept of Qi in the Guanzi's Four Daoist Chapters
– John Cheng*

Here are two additional translations of the verse containing
Ling Chi – Reiki 靈氣 from the Nei-Ye:

*It is ever so that man's life is certain to depend on his being
content. Through sorrow he loses his guiding thread; through
anger he loses his beginnings. In sorrow and melancholy, joy and
anger. The Way can find no resting place. Love and desires – quiet
them. Stupidity and confusion – rectify them. Do not pull. Do
not push. Happiness will naturally be restored. That the Way will
naturally comes. Is something you can count on and plan for. If
you are quiescent, you will obtain it. If you move hastily, you will
lose it. The spiritual force [ling chi] within the mind, sometimes
arrives and sometimes departs. So fine that nothing can exist
within it; so large that nothing can exist beyond it. The reason we
lose it is because haste is harmful. When the mind is able to retain
a state of quiescence, The Way will naturally become stable. For
the man who comprehends the Way, The lines (of his face) effuse (a
sense of harmony) and his hair exudes it. Within his breast there
is nothing corrupt. Since he practices this method of moderating
desires, nothing ever can cause him harm.*
*– Guanzi: Political, Economic, and Philosophical Essays from
Early China – Edited and translated by W. Allyn Rickett*

*Always – at the birth of people – They certainly have joy. When
they are worried, then they lose these tenets. When they are angry,
then they lose the source. Where there is worry, grief, love, anger,
Then Dao does not dwell. Love and desire: still them. Foolishness
and confusion: properly align them. When you do not pull and do
not push, Good fortune will naturally return to you:
That Dao will naturally arrive, Which you can rely on and
consult with. When you are still, then you attain it, When you*

are impatient, then you lose it. This potent Qi in your mind: One moment it arrives, one moment it departs. It is so tiny there is nothing inside it, It is so great there is nothing outside it. The reason that you lose it. Is because impatience causes harm. When the mind can maintain stillness, Dao will naturally settle there. For people who attain Dao: Regulation supports it and it will not dissipate easily, So that the center in their breast does not fail them. When following the Dao of restraining desire, The ten thousand creatures do not cause harm.

– *Study of Inner Cultivation, translated by Bruce R. Linnell*

And a further note about the word Ling Chi: even though the word Reiki-Ling Chi existed in China in 350-300 BCE, that does not mean that Mikao Usui's system comes from ancient China.

Yes, "Ling Chi" was used in a similar context as "Reiki", to indicate our essence, and also how our mind and internal energy work. But Mikao Usui's system is unique to Mikao Usui. When creating his system to help us realize our True Self, he borrowed specific practices from Japanese esoteric teachings. There are indeed very similar practices around in Japan, as most of teachers of the times borrowed from the same esoteric traditions. But the way they put them together is different and that is why Mikao Usui's system is unique. So as we practice Mikao Usui's system of Reiki, we can let go of/transmute our anger and worry. We can regain our "guiding thread", our True Self.

Appendix

To close out and bring together the concepts we have explored, I offer a few additional teachings which you might find helpful to understand the system of Reiki and the journey we are taking towards rediscovering our True Self. These teachings are very important to embody as Reiki practitioners and/or teachers, as they really reflect what Mikao Usui was trying to teach us.

Non-Dual Reiki

Imagine you are sitting on a bench in a park. It's a sunny day. There are trees, a few people walking their dogs, a couple of parents with kids, some insects in the grass, flowers everywhere, you can see a small rock garden...

You sit in meditation on the bench, yet your eyes are open. You see everything and yet there is no attachment to what you see; you are in that open state of mind. At that same time, you feel a deep interconnectedness with everything around you. Reiki, your bright light, flows... Your intent is that everything takes from this deep interconnectedness whatever they want, whatever they may need.

Now, when you see the people in the park, are you going to label the Reiki, the interconnectedness with these people, "human Reiki"? It's very unlikely that you will. And when you see the tree you are not going to label it "tree Reiki," when you see the parents you are not going to label it "parents Reiki," when you see the dogs you are not going to label it "animal Reiki," when you see the kids you are not going to label it "kids Reiki," when you see the grass you are not going to label it "grass Reiki," when you see the insects you are not going to label it "insect Reiki," when you see the rocks you are not going to label it "rock Reiki," and when you see the flowers you are not going to label it "flower Reiki." Are you? I don't imagine you are...

You are also not going to say, "That rock needs a lower vibration than the baby because the rock is just a rock." You are also not going to say, "I am at a higher vibration than that person over there so let me heal them." And you probably also are not going to say, that you "need to channel different vibrations to all the different things you see."

Because if we do that, we label and judge. And if our mind is in a place where we label and judge, we are not in that open state of non-dual empty mind anymore. We have travelled to a place of duality: I/you, tall/small, higher/lower, etc.

So instead of travelling to a narrow place of comparisons, you are just going to be Reiki and stay in that open state of mind of interconnectedness, of emptiness. This is the non-dual state of Reiki in which our open expanded mind feels this deep interconnectedness with all that is, and so everything can benefit from this state of mind. That is the real state of Being Reiki, our True Self. Because when we label and are in this dual mind all the time we are not compassionate, as true compassion comes from our awakened nature of mind, emptiness, non-duality.

In an absolute sense, compassion is the awakened nature of the mind.
– Dilgo Khyentse Rinpoche

As we have seen, the essence of the system of Reiki is all about non-duality. Mikao Usui pointed this out again and again within his system, within the precepts, the symbols and mantras, within the meditation practices, the reiju, and also within hands on/off healing.

The purpose of renunciation mind, compassion, the recitation of mantras, and contemplation on the breath is to dig out dualism. These practices will dismantle the puzzle of dualism.
– Dzongsar Khyentse Rinpoche

When we tap into the deeper layers of the system of Reiki, we slowly start to experience aspects of this non-dual state of mind. This is the ultimate truth. Therefore, as practitioners, we have to focus on this non-duality, because it is in this state of non-duality that we truly can start to heal ourselves.

As we have seen, returning to our foundation, this non-dual state is described within the precepts:

Do not anger
Do not worry
Be grateful
Be true to your way and your being
Show compassion to yourself and others

However, often we find this very difficult, and so we sit in the park and label everything as if that kind of Reiki has a higher vibration than the other. Or we sit in the park with the idea that there are different kinds of Reiki, like "human Reiki" or "tree Reiki" and that they are different from each other. But by doing this we keep focusing on duality, and it is this duality that triggers anger, worry, fear, and keeps us from feeling true compassion. In other words, duality keeps us from embodying the precepts. And when we teach these dual elements to our students, we are guiding our students towards anger, worry and fear, and not towards compassion at all. Without meaning to or without even realizing it, we are guiding our students away from the precepts that we are trying to teach them. This is why it is so important to sit on our butt and practice the meditation practices Mikao Usui put into his system, so that we can start to have insight into this non-dual nature. This in turn will help us to guide our students into the direction of non-duality, true healing. Through doing this we also start to walk a path towards compassion, as is pointed out within the precepts.

Because when we focus on duality in our practice and/or our

teachings (this is better/higher than that, this is different than that), then we carry this through into our daily life. And we might start to say or think things like, "I am going to be kind and supportive of this group but not of that group," "I only like these kinds of people and not those," "I am a better practitioner than you because I use a higher vibration," "I am better than you because I work with humans, animals or trees." So as you can see, duality triggers division; division triggers anger, worry, and fear and not compassion. Non-duality triggers compassion.

If we are missing nonduality, our every act will lead to disappointment.

– Dzongsar Khyentse Rinpoche

As Mikao Usui based his teachings on non-duality, it is therefore important that we are not embracing or straying into dualism in our practice and teachings. Because in essence we all want a peaceful, compassionate world and this peaceful compassion can only manifest when we lay bare our non-dual nature.

If you don't try to better yourself daily, you will easily be led astray. If you don't cultivate your practice daily, it will rust. So here you must not lose track of your True Self, and [you must] attain Buddhahood every day. You have to approach your food as if you were attaining Buddhahood. In all situations, never lose sight of the True Self.

– Discovering the True Self by Kōdō Sawaki

Self-Responsibility

You are holding a cup of coffee when someone comes along and shoves you or shakes your arm, making you spill your coffee everywhere. "Why did you spill the coffee?" "Well because someone bumped into me, of course!" Wrong answer. You spilled the coffee because coffee was in the cup. If tea had been in it, you would have spilled tea. Whatever is inside the cup is what will come out. Therefore, when life comes along and shakes you (which will happen), whatever is inside of you will come out. It's easy to fake it until you get rattled. So we have to ask ourselves... what's in my cup? When life gets tough, what spills over? Joy, gratefulness, peace and humility? Or anger, bitterness, harsh words and actions?

– author unknown

When we walk through life, many people will bump us or shake us; we cannot avoid this. But we have the power to change our reaction to it when people or situations bump or shake us. We have the power to change what is inside us. Most of the time we start to blame others: you made me angry, you did that or this to me. Blaming others is much easier to do because if we want to change our reactions, to change what is in the cup so to speak, we need to step into that space of self-responsibility.

Self-responsibility is taking a step towards healing ourselves, towards empowering ourselves. But this takes time and practice. The practice part means to start doing some self-inquiry about why we are holding on to the anger, why we are bitter or harsh. It means looking at our own issues, bringing up our anger and bitterness so that we can soften them and maybe one day transform them into joy, love, and gratefulness.

So if you feel hatred, stand up straight and face your hatred. Accept it, deal with it as simply as you can, and then let it go. Let your hatred and you return to emptiness together. That's all you can do. In the next moment that form of hatred is gone, and something new is arising. Whatever it is, accept it, and be free from it. Just keep walking step by step.

– The Light That Shines Through Infinity by Dainin Katagiri

This transformation can be done in many ways, through many

practices. Meditation practice is one of my own favorite ways, as it helps us to rest our mind so that we can look very clearly at our anger and bitterness. In that quiet space of meditation we can slowly let go of our grasping of the past, present, and future. This kind of letting go is needed to empty our cup. The more we grasp at the past, present, and future, the more we hold all our anger and bitterness in our cup, there will be no way to empty it. Thus whenever someone bumps us, we will spill anger and bitterness instead of gratitude and love.

Self-responsibility is therefore about looking within instead of looking outside of yourself, blaming others. So take that step towards self-responsibility and let go of the anger and bitterness in your cup. Start practicing meditation practices so that you can transform that anger and bitterness into gratitude and love. So the next time someone bumps or shakes you, gratitude and love spill out.

When you think everything is someone else's fault, you will suffer a lot.
– 14th Dalai Lama

Blaming

People who blame others have a long way to go on their journey. People who blame themselves are halfway there. A person who blames no one has arrived.
– Chinese proverb

In this day and age there is so much blaming going on. Women blame men and men blame women, people blame governments and governments blame people, husbands blame wives and wives blame husbands, students blame teachers and teachers blame students, we blame nature and nature... oh hang on... nature is just nature, it is not blaming anybody. As we are nature ourselves, we need to learn how to let go of blaming and take self-responsibility. Self-responsibility can help us to grow and blossom, to be like nature, as this is what we really are. Self-responsibility is about empowering ourselves, standing on our own two feet, living fully in the present moment. Blaming, on the other hand, is often focused on the past. But the past is past; let it go. That doesn't mean we have to be okay with what has happened in the past, but we need to learn how to let go. If we keep pointing our fingers at others, we are in fact losing our own self-responsibility and hence we are disempowering ourselves. Plus by blaming others we place ourselves in the role of the sufferer, and the more we blame the more we suffer.

But how do we take self-responsibility? We can do that through coming back to our self, back to our own center, our inner light. This we can do through internalizing practices like meditation, yoga, tai chi and so on. Self-responsibility is not an easy path and that is why so many people instead put the blame on other people or on external factors. This may be much easier to do, but in reality it is very disempowering. So let's take the step, go inwards, and rediscover our own innate power through practices like meditation so that we can take full self-responsibility. In that way, we can let things go and be free, free from suffering.

The next time you lose heart and you can't bear to experience what you're feeling, you might recall this instruction: change the way you see it and lean in. Instead of blaming our discomfort on outer circumstances or on our own weakness, we can choose to stay present and awake to our experience, not rejecting it, not grasping it, not buying the stories that we relentlessly tell ourselves. This is priceless advice that addresses the true cause of suffering – yours, mine, and that of all living beings.
– Pema Chödrön

Together in Harmony

You and everything in the universe, without exception, are travelling together. We are all passengers in one big boat – the universal boat. This is the original state of everyone's existence. That's why we have to walk together, hand in hand, and make an effort to live together in peace and harmony.
– The Light That Shines Through Infinity by Dainin Katagiri

In 2019 I spent five days at the 35th Northwest Reiki Gathering in Oregon, USA where I was asked to be one of the guest speakers. The other two speakers were Paul Mitchell, who is the head of discipline for Usui Shiki Ryôhô, and Hyakuten Inamoto, the founder of Kômyô ReikiDo.

As the theme of this conference was "Being Together in the Harmony of Reiki", it was a unique opportunity to learn and share teachings from different traditions.

What was so wonderful about this gathering is that it gave the opportunity to listen to each of the speakers without thinking about one system being better than the other, or that we need to be in conflict or competition with one another. It was an opportunity to grow, to be open without judgements, to share and to explore different viewpoints.

This of course is not always easy and that is okay. We all have our own ideas, beliefs, and patterns that we hold on to and often we take for granted. But when sitting in that space of openness and non-judgement, we are in fact expanding our own mind. And therefore the Reiki will flow much more deeply and brightly.

Of course we don't all have to agree and that is fine too. But we can hold hands and support each other in each other's journey, because that is really what the system of Reiki is all about.

The teacher is not there to impose their teachings onto a

student, or anyone. The teacher is there to create a space in which the student can remember that they are Reiki, their inner great bright light. And this state of great bright light is called spiritual freedom, being free from spiritual dogma.

During one of the discussion sessions, about 90 people paired up in small groups, I sat in meditation and could also see Paul Mitchell sitting in meditation to hold the space for everybody. At that moment I felt a deep interconnectedness with him and a clear thought surfaced from this interconnectedness state of mind. This thought was that at that moment Paul and I were supporting each other to go deeper into our True Self, our great bright light, without the need to impose the idea that he should start following and teaching my way or that I should start following and teaching his way. Just helping each other to go deeper into our own way without imposing something on the other: a state of pure love and compassion. This space touched me deeply and triggered an amazing state of love for him, a love without asking anything in return, a love of holding each other in an open hand, pure love.

I had many other wonderful experiences during this retreat, not just during the teachings and hands on healing sessions but also just having breakfast with people or laughing together or bathing in one of the amazing hot springs.

Most people who used the hot springs sat in it naked, but you could also wear a bathing suit or swimmers. At one stage I sat in one of the hot springs together with a woman, who had one breast removed due to cancer, and a man with one leg who also was deaf. We sat there being naked with each other, not just on a physical level but naked with all our issues, nowhere to hide. This experience was so sobering; we all have issues and scars, either physical or emotional. To share them in such an open way was very profound.

Many people are afraid of their physical nakedness. Or afraid of being truly naked with someone, not physically naked, but without the invisible masks so many of us wear. But when we start to practice the system of Reiki, we start to make friends again with our physical body, and this in turn also helps us to start to drop our masks. When we do this, we can be in a state of nakedness with our mind/heart.

So even though I was the speaker – the teacher, so to speak – I also was the student. We cannot divide those two; we learn so much when we start to realize this, that we are the student and the teacher at the same time.

But to be able to learn during conferences, retreats and gatherings like this, we have to enter them with an open mind. If our mind is full of judgement and fixed ideas we cannot learn; we are not empty enough to learn. Just like we cannot fill a cup of tea which is already full.

I hope that more and more people start to see that as a Reiki community we need to hold hands, to look at the similarities instead of the differences. Because it is only in this way that the world will become a better place for all.

As one human being, if you want the human world as a whole to develop, you have to take responsibility and do something. Life is depending on you to act. What should you do? Open your heart, live mindfully, and start to walk with all beings. That way of walking is steadfast, tranquil, and positive. You share your life and practice benevolence, and compassion. This is the practice of walking alone with an open heart.

– The Light That Shines Through Infinity by Dainin Katagiri

Glossary of Japanese Terms

Anshin Ritsumei – spiritual peace in our mind, enlightenment
Choku Rei – True Self, direct or straight spirit
Dai Ajari – great esoteric master
Dai Kômyô – great bright light, void, non-duality, emptiness
Gakkai – society
Gassho – putting your palms together, union, non-duality
Gyō – practice, ascetic practices
Hara – stomach, center, true center, center of our True Self
Hatsurei-hō – a method to emanate a greater amount of spirit
Hō – Dharma, method, truth, teachings
Hon sha ze sho nen – I am Right Mind, my original nature is a
    non-dual thought
Jōshin – focusing the mind
Kaji – the transference of the Buddha's power or grace which
    inspires a sacred peace of mind and a strengthening of the
    life force
Ki – energy, breath, air, life force
Kokyū – breathing, in and out breath
Ku – emptiness, void
Okuden – hidden or inner teachings
Reiju – spiritual blessing, spiritual offering
Reiki – True Self, spiritual energy
Ryô – to cure, to heal
Sanmitsu – three mysteries of mind, body, and speech/energy/
    breath
Satori – enlightenment
Sei heki – inclination to remember our True Self
Shinpiden – mystery teachings, not just for teaching but for
    deepening your personal practice, remembering the
    mystery of the universe and life
Shoden – beginner's teachings

Tanden – field of elixir, ocean of ki
Toitsu – to unite, to unify

Bibliography

Addiss, Stephen. *Zen Sourcebook: Traditional Documents from China, Korea, and Japan*. Indianapolis: Hackett Publishing Company, 2008.

Ahn, Juhn Y. *Worms, Germs, and Technologies of the Self – Religion, Sword Fighting, and Medicine in Early Modern Japan*. Essay, 2012.

Boutry-Stadelmann, Britta. *Yuasa Yasuo's Theory of the Body*. Essay, 2008.

Bowring, Richard. *The Religious Traditions of Japan 500-1600*. Port Melbourne: Cambridge University Press, 2008.

Breen, John and Mark Teeuwen. *Shinto in History: Ways of the Kami*. Surrey: Curzon Press, 2000.

Carter, Robert E. *The Japanese Arts and Self-Cultivation*. State University of New York Press, 2007.

Cheng, John. *Re-figuring St. Thomas's Concept of Ipsum Esse Subsistens in terms of the Concept of Qi in the Guanzi's Four Daoist Chapters*. Essay, 2013.

Chowang, Orgyen. *Our Pristine Mind: A Practical Guide to Unconditional Happiness*. Shambhala Publications, Inc., 2016.

Cleary, Thomas. *Code of the Samurai: A Modern Translation of the Bushido Shoshinshu of Taira Shigesuke*. Boston: Tuttle Publishing, 2000.

Cleary, Thomas. *Zen Essence: The Science of Freedom*, Shambhala Dragon Edition. Boston: Shambhala Publications, 2000.

Davey, H.E. *The Japanese Way of the Artist*. Albany, CA: Michi Publishing, 2015.

Davey, H.E. *The Teachings of Tempu: Practical Meditation for Daily Life*. Albany, CA: Michi Publishing, 2013.

Deshimaru, Taisen. *Mushotoku Mind: The Heart of the Heart Sutra*. Chino Valley: Hohm Press, 2012.

Doi, Hiroshi. *A Modern Reiki Method for Healing*. Southfield:

Vision Publications, 2014.

Eidson, Eijun. What is Kaji. *Lion's Roar – Buddhist Wisdom for Our Time*, 2004.

Gleason, William. *Aikido and Words of Power: The Sacred Sounds of Kototama*. Rochester: Destiny Books, 2009.

Gleason, William. *The Spiritual Foundations of Aikido*. Rochester: Destiny Books, 1995.

Goi, Masahisa. *God and Man: Guideposts for Spiritual Peace and Awakening*. Japan: Byakko Press, 2002.

Goi, Masahisa. *Living Like the Blue Sky: five talks by Masahisa Goi*. Japan: Byakko Press, 2015.

Gray, John Harvey. *Hand to Hand*. Xlibris, 2002.

Groner, Paul. *Saicho: The Establishment of the Japanese Tendai School*. Honolulu: University of Hawaii Press, 2000.

Hakeda, Yoshito S. *Kukai: Major Works*. New York: Columbia University Press, 1972.

Hanh, Thich Nhat. *True Love: A Practice for Awakening the Heart*. Boston: Shambhala Publications, 2004.

Harada, Shodo. Ten Ox Herding Pictures, public talk, 1998.

Herrigel, Eugen. *Zen in the Art of Archery*. London: Vintage, 1999.

Hitoshi, Miyake. *The Mandala of the Mountain: Shugendo and Folk Religion*. Tokyo: Keio University Press Inc., 2005.

Hitoshi, Miyake. *Shugendo: Essays on the Structure of Japanese Folk Religion*. The University of Michigan, 2001.

Hyers, Conrad. *Once-Born, Twice-Born Zen: The Soto and Rinzai Schools of Japan*. Eugene: WIPF & Stock Publishing, 2004.

Inagaki, Hisao. *A Dictionary of Japanese Buddhist Terms*. Kyoto: Nagata Bunshodo, 2003.

Japanese Journals of Religious Studies. Japan: Nanzan Institute for Religion and Culture.

Kalu, Rinpoche. *Luminous Mind*. Wisdom Publications, 1993.

Kamalashila. *Meditation: The Buddhist Way of Tranquility and Insight*. Glasgow: Windhorse Publications, 1992.

Katagiri, Dainin. *Each Moment is the Universe: Zen and the Way of*

Being Time. Boston: Shambhala Publications, 2007.

Katagiri, Dainin. *The Light That Shines Through Infinity*. Boston: Shambhala Publications, 2017.

Katagiri, Dainin. *You Have to Say Something: Manifesting Zen Insight*. Boston: Shambhala Publications, 2000.

Kohno, Jiko. *Right View, Right Life: Insights of a Woman Buddhist Priest*. Tokyo: Kosei Publishing Co., 1998.

Kukai. *Shingon Texts*. Moraga, CA: Numata Center for Buddhist Translation & Research, 2004.

Kwong, Jakusho. *No Beginning, No End: The Intimate Heart of Zen*. Boston: Shambhala Publications, 2003.

Leyi, Li. *Evolutionary Illustration of Chinese Characters*. Beijing Language and Culture University Press, 2000.

Leyi, Li. *Tracing the Roots of Chinese Characters*. Beijing Language and Culture University Press, 1997.

Linnell, Bruce R. *Study of Inner Cultivation*. Essay, 2012.

Low, Albert. *Hakuin on Kensho*. Boston: Shambhala Publications, 2006.

Maezumi, Taizan. *Appreciate Your Life: The Essence of Zen Practice*. Boston: Shambhala Publications, 2002.

Maltese, Maurizio. *Zen and the Art of Self Preservation: The strategies of the martial arts servicing your life*. Milan: Carabá Publishing House, 2014.

Mitchell, Damo. *A Comprehensive Guide to Daoist Nei Gong*. Singing Dragon, 2018.

Mitchell, Stephen. *The Tao Te Ching: a new English version*. Harper Perennial Modern Classics, 2006.

Morinaga, Soko. *Novice to Master: An Ongoing Lesson in The Extent of My Own Stupidity*. Somerville: Wisdom Publications, 2002.

Myodo, Satomi. *Passionate Journey: The Spiritual Autobiography of Satomi Myodo*. Boston: Shambhala Publications, 1987.

Nakazono, Masahilo. *Inochi: The Book of Life*. Kototama Institute; Revised edition, 1984.

Nakazono, Masahilo. *My Past Way of Budo*. Kototama Institute, 2002.

Oda, Ryuko. *Kaji: Empowerment and Healing in Esoteric Buddhism*. Japan: Kineizan Shinjo-in Mitsumonkai, 1992.

Picken, Stuart D.B. *Essentials of Shinto: An Analytical Guide to Principal Teachings*. Greenwood, 1994.

Reid, Daniel. *Harnessing the Power of the Universe: A Complete Guide to the Principles and Practice of Chi-Gung*. Boston: Shambhala Publications, 1998.

Rickett, W. Allyn. *Guanzi: Political, Economic, and Philosophical Essays from Early China*. Princeton University Press, 1998.

Saotome, Mitsugi. *Principles of Aikido*. Boston: Shambhala Publications, 1989.

Saso, Michael. *Tantric Art and Meditation: Tendai Tradition*. Honolulu: Education Foundation, 1990.

Sawaki, Kōdō. *Discovering the True Self*. Counterpoint, 2020.

Shaner, David Edward. *The Bodymind Experience in Japanese Buddhism: A Phenomenological Perspective of Kukai and Dogen*. Albany: State University of New York Press, 1985.

Shionuma, Ryōjun. *The Life-long Spiritual Journey of an Apprentice Japanese Bonze: Awakening to a new worldview by fulfilling the One-thousand Days Trekking Practice on Mt. Ōmine*. Tokyo: Pro Sophia, 2014.

Smart, Ninian. *World Philosophies*. New York: Routledge, 2008.

Sogen, Omori. *Introduction to Zen Training: A Physical Approach to Meditation and Mind-Body Training*. Tuttle Publishing, 2020.

Soho, Takuan. *The Unfettered Mind: Writings of the Zen Master to a Master Swordsman*. Tokyo: Kodansha International, 1986.

Stevens, John. *The Heart of Aikido: The Philosophy of Takemusu Aiki by Morihei Ueshiba*. Tokyo: Kodansha International Ltd., 2010.

Stevens, John. *The Philosophy of Aikido*. Echo Point Books & Media, 2013.

Stevens, John. *Sacred Calligraphy of the East*. Routledge, 1996.

Stevens, John. *The Secrets of Aikido*. Shambhala, 1997.

Stiene, Bronwen and Frans. *A–Z of Reiki Pocketbook: Everything About Reiki*. Winchester: O-Books, 2006.

Stiene, Bronwen and Frans. *The Japanese Art of Reiki*. Winchester: O-Books, 2005.

Stiene, Bronwen and Frans. *The Reiki Sourcebook*. Winchester: O-Books, 2003.

Stiene, Bronwen and Frans. *Your Reiki Treatment*. Winchester: O-Books, 2007.

Stiene, Frans. *The Inner Heart of Reiki: Rediscovering Your True Self*. Hants: Ayni Books, 2015.

Stiene, Frans. *Reiki Insights*. Hants: Anyi Books, 2018.

Stone, Jacqueline. *Original Enlightenment and the Transformation of Medieval Japanese Buddhism*. Honolulu: University of Hawaii Press, 2003.

Suzuki, Shunryu. *Branching Streams Flow in the Darkness: Zen Talks on the Sandokai*. Berkeley: University of California Press, 1999.

Suzuki, Shunryu. *Not Always So: Practicing the True Spirit of Zen*. New York: Harper Collins, 2002.

Suzuki, Shunryu. *Zen Mind, Beginner's Mind.* New York: Weatherhill, 1970.

Tachikawa, Musashi. *Buddhist Fire Ritual in Japan*. Osaka: National Museum of Ethnology, 2012.

Tanabe, George J., Jr. *Religions of Japan in Practice*. Princeton: Princeton University Press, 1999.

Tarthang Tulku. *Openness Mind: Self-Knowledge and Inner Peace Through Meditation*. Cazadero: Dharma Publishing, 1990.

Thrangu, Khenchen. *Medicine Buddha Teachings*. Snow Lion, 2004.

Thrangu, Khenchen. *The Practice of Tranquillity and Insight*. Boston: Shambhala Publications, 1993.

Tohei, Koichi. *Aikido: The Co-ordination of Mind and Body for Self-*

defence. Souvenir Press, 1996.

Tohei, Koichi. *Book of Ki: Co-ordinating Mind and Body in Daily Life.* Tokyo: Japan Publications Inc., 1976.

Tohei, Koichi. *Ki in Daily Life.* Tokyo: Ki-no-Kenkyukai, 1980.

Ueshiba, Morihei. *The Art of Peace.* Boston: Shambhala Publications, 2002.

Unno, Taitetsu. *Shin Buddhism: Bits of Rubble Turn into Gold.* Image, 2002.

Urgyen, Tulku. *As It Is.* Rangjung Yeshe Publications, 1999.

Waddell, Norman. *Hakuin's Precious Mirror Cave.* Berkeley: Counterpoint, 2009.

Wilson, William Scott. *The Demon's Sermon on the Martial Arts.* Tokyo: Kodansha International, 2006.

Wilson, William Scott. *The Swordsman's Handbook: Samurai Teachings on the Path of the Sword.* Boston: Shambhala Publications, 2014.

Wilson, William Scott. *The Unfettered Mind.* Tokyo: Kodansha International, 1986.

Wilson, William Scott. *Yojokun: Life Lessons from a Samurai.* Tokyo: Kodansha International, 2009.

Wong, Eva. *Cultivating Stillness: A Taoist Manual for Transforming Body and Mind.* Boston: Shambhala Publications, 1992.

Yamakage, Motohisa. *The Essence of Shinto: Japan's Spiritual Heart.* Tokyo: Kodansha International, 2006.

Yamaoka, Seigen. *The Art and the Way of Hara.* Heian International, 1998.

Yamasaki, Taiko. *Shingon: Japanese Esoteric Buddhism.* Boston: Shambhala Publications, 1988.

Yasuo, Yuasa. *The Body, Self-Cultivation, and Ki-Energy.* Albany: State University of New York Press, 1993.

Yen, Sheng. *Attaining the Way: A Guide to the Practice of Chan Buddhism.* Boston: Shambhala Publications, 2006.

Yeshe, Lama Thubten. *When the Chocolate Runs Out.* Somerville: Wisdom Publications, 2011.

Yuho, Tseng. *A History of Chinese Calligraphy*. The Chinese University Press, 1993.

Who is Frans Stiene?

Frans has been a major influence on global research into the system of Reiki since the early 2000s. His practical understanding of the Japanese influences on the system has allowed students around the world to connect deeply with this practice. Students naturally respond to Frans' warmth and intelligence. His own personal spiritual practice is a model that many students wish to emulate, and offers great encouragement to those on the same path. Frans is a co-founder of the International House of Reiki and Shibumi International Reiki Association with Bronwen Logan (Stiene). He has also coauthored with her the critically acclaimed books *The Reiki Sourcebook*, *The Japanese Art of Reiki*, *A–Z of Reiki Pocketbook*, *Reiki Techniques Card Deck* and *Your Reiki Treatment*. He himself wrote the popular Reiki books, *The Inner Heart of Reiki: Rediscovering Your True Self*, and *Reiki Insights*. His books have been translated into numerous languages.

Frans is based in Holland, and since 1998 he has trained in a variety of countries such as Japan, Nepal, Italy, UK and Australia. Some of his Reiki teachers include Hyakuten Inamoto, Doi Hiroshi and Chris Marsh. Frans' research has included interviewing Chiyoko Yamaguchi and other Japanese teachers, including Dr. Matsuoka. Although Frans is trained as a Gendai Reiki Ho Shihan (teacher) and a Kômyô Reiki Shihan (teacher), he prefers to teach a traditional form of Japanese Reiki, Usui Reiki Ryôhô, that he feels reflects a desire to bring the teachings back to their very source, rediscovering our True Self.

Most teachers in Japan teach the system of Reiki from Chujiro Hayashi's viewpoint while Frans tries to teach it as much as possible from Mikao Usui's viewpoint.

To learn more about Shinto, Shugendo, Tendai, and Shingon, Frans is currently training with Japanese Shingon priest Takeda

Hakusai Ajari, who was once a Tendai monk as a disciple of the great Sakai Dai Ajari. In 2019, Frans took a group of his students to Japan to meet with Takeda Hakusai Ajari for teachings and training.

Frans keeps researching and practicing traditional Japanese teachings to find out what Mikao Usui himself was practicing to get a deeper understanding about what the system of Reiki is really about. This will help him to become a better teacher and to support students in their understanding of the system and their own personal spiritual practice. Frans is one of the rare Reiki teachers who is undertaking these practices.

– Reverend Kûban Jakkôin, Shugendo priest

The contents of what Frans teaches is formed by what has been practiced in Japan since the early 1900s, long before the system of Reiki left Japan, and the researched influences on the system. This particular method includes physical and energy-enhancing exercises to help practitioners delve deeper into their Reiki practice. The earlier teachings consider the system not just to be a hands-on-healing practice but one that also focuses on a student's spiritual path.

The spiritual level of the practitioner directly reflects the effect of Reiki. In a sense, the more you are enlightened, the more the effectiveness of Reiki enhances. The more you practice Reiki for saving others, the brighter your innate light shines to drive away clouds covering your mind. I think this is the quintessence of Reiki. I hope Frans Stiene's way of understanding Reiki spreads in the world to enlighten those who practice Reiki based on a superficial understanding of the tradition.

– Reverend Takeda Hakusai

Frans' open, humorous, and informal style of teaching has been an inspiration for students and clients throughout the USA, Europe, Asia, and Australia. His aim is to provide students with the most comprehensive and up-to-date information about the system of Reiki as well as a strong energetic connection to Mikao Usui's teachings.

Apart from teaching all three levels of the system of Reiki and specialized classes, Frans offers limited one-on-one training sessions for students and one hour hands on/off healing sessions all over the word. He also does one-on-one Skype sessions, teaches through teleclasses, and offers retreats. During his retreats, students delve deep into rediscovering their True Self, which is a must for Reiki practitioners who want to help others. His Shinpiden Reiki III courses are attended by many existing Reiki teachers who want to take their practice to a deeper level.

For more information on courses, blogs and more, visit the International House of Reiki website:

www.IHReiki.com
International House of Reiki on Facebook: www.facebook.com/IHReiki
Frans Stiene on Facebook: https://www.facebook.com/frans.stiene
Frans Stiene on Instagram: https://www.instagram.com/stienefrans/

What people are saying about

The Inner Heart of Reiki:
Rediscovering Your True Self:

I am a Tendai monk, the founder of Tendai Sect, Denkyo Daishi Saicho, which stresses Doshin – Heart for the Way – as of most importance. In Denjyutsu Isshin Kaimon, Kojo (Tendai monk, 779-858) quotes Saicho's famous words: "There is livelihood in Doshin, there is Doshin in livelihood." I had the opportunity to spend a week with Frans Stiene upon his visit to Japan, when I had the honor of guiding him through Buddhist practices. I was thoroughly impressed with Frans' Doshin and was struck with awe. In high regards to Frans Stiene's Doshin, I have presented him with the Kesa – monk's stole – which I received upon initiation to priesthood. Kesa is the soul of a priest. Having witnessed his Doshin and soul, both in person and through *The Inner Heart of Reiki: Rediscovering Your True Self*, I look forward to Frans' further endeavors. Reiki is not merely a "technique", but has a vital role in guiding one to reach "perfection as a human being". The idea contained in the precepts, "Just for today, do not anger, do not worry..." also is reflected in One Day, One Life by my teacher, Sakai Yusai Dai Ajari. If you want to know whether a teacher is a true Reiki teacher or not, all you have to do is to ask him what the True Self is. Without the trustworthy insight of the True Self, nobody can insist he or she is a true disciple of Mikao Usui. This book testifies that the author is one of the true Reiki teachers.
– Takeda Hakusai Ajari

The Inner Heart of Reiki resonated deeply within me, for I have always believed that we are all one and that Oneness is the essence of our universe. In this book Frans Stiene takes us on a journey through Japanese Buddhist teachings and meanings of mantras and kanji as taught by Mikao Usui. It is a journey back to our True Self, Oneness and being Reiki rather than living in duality and just doing Reiki. This book is a must-read not just for Reiki Practitioners and Teachers but for everyone who is on life's journey of discovery. So much of Frans' research, study, and practice are openly shared with the reader. Frans does not just talk the talk; he genuinely walks the walk.

The Australian Reiki Connection Inc. is pleased to endorse *The Inner Heart of Reiki* to its members and to the Reiki community.
– **John Coleman**, president of Australian Reiki Connection Inc., Australia's leading Reiki association

Every once in a while you find a book that changes everything. It is almost like you have a paradigm shift, and you take the words into your new understanding of how the world could be. Things that you always questioned come clearer even though you did not know that there was confusion. Frans Stiene's new book *The Inner Heart of Reiki* is just such a book. Every page took me deeper into myself and lit up the places where there were shadows of doubt about the system of Reiki and the spiritual path that I am on. I have studied Buddhism for a number of years and have been working on becoming a Zen priest for the past few years. I also have a yoga studio and have trained in yoga for the past 20 years. Neither Zen nor yoga have been able to take me as close to my true nature as Reiki has done. When asked what religion I am, I say I am a Reiki Buddhist for that reason. In Buddhism there is a well-renowned sutra called the Diamond Sutra. It is called the Diamond Sutra because it cuts through delusion. This book is similar in that it cuts through the delusion and hype of typical Reiki books and goes right to the core of what Reiki really is, a spiritual path. This book hits the mark and the mark, it turns out, is the true self. Frans has gone further than anyone in the world to study and learn about the system of Reiki and it shows on every page, always bringing us back to our True Self, inviting readers to explore for themselves what the true essence is all about. We are fortunate that Frans has done the research for us and we can all follow the path that he has cleared for us. I have decided that I will not teach anyone the third level of Reiki unless they have read this book, because if they have not we cannot have a good conversation of what the deeper elements of the system of Reiki are, so there would be no reason to advance anyone to that level.

– **Jeff Emerson**, author of *Unfolding the Lotus*

This is a must-read for all students of the system of Reiki. Frans, through his research and practice, has peeled away the myths about the system of Reiki and gives us a clear understanding of the Reiki journey. He also shows how meditation practice is a fundamental part of the system. This book is just what the Reiki world needs, written by someone who walks his talk.

– **Helen Galpin**, co-founder of the British School of Meditation

Having investigated The Great Way of the Asians in shamanism, Daoism, Buddhism, medicine, ancient science, Tai Chi and Qigong since 1963-4, I have a special appreciation of any "system" that articulates the natural presence of the truth and power of the Universe within a context of Self. Versions of self-discovery, self-awareness, ultimate personal potential and the revelation of the True Self – from Lao Zi and Daoists, to Shakyamuni and the Buddhist flourishing, to the great Zen monks and poets – all point to the same views, insights and practices. Mikao Usui's Way is one of those beautiful articulations of the mastery of the nature of human experience and the True Self. Frans Stiene has done us a huge favor by revealing the actual context of Reiki as a Way of Self-Cultivation which is primarily focused on refinement of self which happens to include a method of helping and healing others that is a secondary feature of The Way.

– **Dr. Roger Jahnke**, OMD, founder/director of the Institute of Integral Qigong and Tai Chi (IIQTC); author of *The Healer Within* and *The Healing Promise of Qi*

Frans Stiene is an inspiring teacher because he embodies the spiritual gift of Reiki in all his actions and throughout his day, not just when giving someone a session. In this delightful book he weaves the threads of the rich history of Japanese spiritual practices that have brought him to this inner sacred space.
– **Neil McKinney**, MD, author of *Naturopathic Oncology*

Frans Stiene illuminates the intricacies of Reiki with the insight and simple elegance of a master. His writing resonates with the depth of experience.
– **Barry Lancet**, award-winning author of *Japantown*

What people are saying about

Reiki Insights:

This profound and powerful book illuminates our understanding of the true nature of Reiki. Frans Stiene, one of the world's leading Reiki Teachers, takes us on a journey to the heart of Reiki and unwraps its power to transform and heal.
– **Mary Pearson**, author, *Meditation: The Stress Solution*

From a holistic nursing perspective, *Reiki Insights* is an exceptional read for all Reiki practitioners working in the field of healthcare. Each concise chapter is a gentle reminder of how we can embody the precepts in order to live in a compassionate and mindful way. Nurturing compassion within ourselves is the key to avoiding burnout in a healthcare system that is often fraught with stress and worry. Frans Stiene, a phenomenal teacher and author, has once again given us a beautiful gift which lovingly guides us on our path to be true to our way and our being.
– **Helene Williams**, BSN, RN, Reiki Teacher/Hospital & Hospice Practitioner, Founder and President, Lancaster Community Reiki Clinic

With *Reiki Insights*, world-renowned Reiki teacher Frans Stiene offers yet another gift to the world... and not just to the world of Reiki. He takes us through a journey that takes us back to the beginning, through the end and the middle, to the insight of who we truly are. For Reiki practitioners and seekers, yes, but also for seekers who are being called back into the heart of the matter, this book will help us to reach and touch into who we really are.
– **Kathryn Hudson**, author of *The Angels Told Me So: Practical guide for lightworkers*

Most of us have only a superficial understanding of the system of Reiki. In this extraordinary work *Reiki Insights*, Frans Stiene, one of the godfathers of Reiki in the West, reveals the system of Reiki to be not only a method of healing, but nothing less than a pathway to enlightenment. If you have ever wanted to explore the deeper meaning of the system of Reiki, this illuminating treasure is for you!

– **David Michie**, author of *The Dalai Lama's Cat* Series

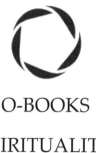

O-BOOKS

SPIRITUALITY

O is a symbol of the world, of oneness and unity; this eye
represents knowledge and insight. We publish titles on general
spirituality and living a spiritual life. We aim to inform and help
you on your own journey in this life.
If you have enjoyed this book, why not tell other readers by
posting a review on your preferred book site?

Recent bestsellers from O-Books are:

Heart of Tantric Sex
Diana Richardson
Revealing Eastern secrets of deep love and intimacy to Western
couples.
Paperback: 978-1-90381-637-0 ebook: 978-1-84694-637-0

Crystal Prescriptions
The A-Z guide to over 1,200 symptoms and their healing crystals
Judy Hall
The first in the popular series of eight books, this handy little
guide is packed as tight as a pill-bottle with crystal remedies for
ailments.
Paperback: 978-1-90504-740-6 ebook: 978-1-84694-629-5

Take Me To Truth
Undoing the Ego
Nouk Sanchez, Tomas Vieira
The best-selling step-by-step book on shedding the Ego, using the
teachings of *A Course In Miracles.*
Paperback: 978-1-84694-050-7 ebook: 978-1-84694-654-7

The 7 Myths about Love...Actually!
The Journey from your HEAD to the HEART of your SOUL
Mike George
Smashes all the myths about LOVE.
Paperback: 978-1-84694-288-4 ebook: 978-1-84694-682-0

Your Simple Path
Find Happiness in every step
Ian Tucker
A guide to helping us reconnect with what is really important in
our lives.
Paperback: 978-1-78279-349-6 ebook: 978-1-78279-348-9

Readers of ebooks can buy or view any of these bestsellers by
clicking on the live link in the title. Most titles are published
in paperback and as an ebook. Paperbacks are available in
traditional bookshops. Both print and ebook formats are
available online.
Find more titles and sign up to our readers' newsletter at
http://www.johnhuntpublishing.com/mind-body-spirit
Follow us on Facebook at https://www.facebook.com/OBooks/
and Twitter at https://twitter.com/obooks